Praise for David Kahn . . .

"Having served as a Navy SEAL for more than twenty-five years, I recognized premier training when we did it. *This* is krav maga delivered at its highest level—a phenomenal force multiplier. David provides instinctive, simple, and brutally efficient tools to prevail in a violent kinetic or nonkinetic hand-to-hand combat situation. The professional insights and tactics David presents are dead-on serious and practical—no nonsense. I, and other like-minded professionals, continue to train with David. I highly recommend David Kahn's reality-based krav maga approach to everyone who is serious about developing a hand-to-hand capability."

—**S.M., (ret.) Senior Chief Petty Officer**, United States Navy

"On behalf of the Marine Corps Martial Arts Center of Excellence (MACE) I would like to extend my appreciation to David B. Kahn and H. C. 'Sparky' Bollinger, Maj USMC (ret.) as well as their professional training team. On several occasions they have trained the top-level Marine Corps Martial Arts Program (MCMAP) instructor-trainers as well as instructors of the FBI and DEA academy at our facility. Their clear and concise instruction in military hand-to-hand combat, as well as in law enforcement defensive tactics, is of the highest caliber."

—**Lt. Col. (ret.) J. C. Shusko**, United States Marine Corps

"I would like to thank you for providing your expert instruction. . . . This represents an ongoing relationship with the goal of providing top-level best-practices training for all members of law enforcement throughout the state. Based on the response from this course, all agencies involved had nothing but praise for the course and your staff. It is important our tactics continually evolve as new techniques and defensive tactics are developed. I know the academy staff is looking forward to working with you in the future. Your instruction and skill set are at the highest level."

—**Captain S. Munafo**, Commandant, New Jersey State Police
Training Bureau

"I wanted to express my gratitude for the Israeli Krav Maga weapon-defense training that you provided. The opportunity to do these skills 'hands on' with M4, shotgun, as well as the handgun is extremely beneficial. I appreciate that you stuck with real-world tactics and your delivery of the lesson was well taken by the law enforcement audience. Additionally, it was apparent that you are aware of the law enforcement rules of engagement. Thank you also for providing weapon disarming, close quarters/tubular combat, as well as removing subjects from vehicles during [motor vehicle] stops in addition to what you had planned for the day. It is obvious that as the chief instructor of the Israeli Krav Maga Association your knowledge of defensive tactics is extremely beneficial to the law enforcement community."

—**Vladimir Vaval**, New Jersey Transit Police Officer, Training Unit

"I would like to express my gratitude for the training you provided to the officers with the PA Fish and Boat Commission. The Law Enforcement Krav Maga Instructor course was excellent and a true asset to not only my officers but the visiting officers from various departments. The krav maga was effective yet easy to learn and retain, making it very practical for the patrol officer. We look forward to continuing the program and expanding it in the future. Your experience, knowledge of the law, and enthusiasm were greatly appreciated. If the Bureau of Law Enforcement can ever be of assistance in the future, don't hesitate to ask. Thanks again."

> —**Col Corey L. Britcher**, Director, Pennsylvania Bureau
> of Law Enforcement

"I would like to thank you for sharing your expertise in Israeli krav maga with the members of the New Jersey State Police, Executive Protection Bureau. The simplicity of the moves, coupled with effectiveness of the techniques, makes this training useful in real-world situations. I particularly like the disarming training and simultaneous 'block and strike' techniques. Your professional instruction and enthusiastic participation along with you and your entire staff made this training a true success. Israeli krav maga has further prepared the New Jersey State Police, Executive Protection Bureau, in achieving our mission of protecting our principals. We look forward to training with you and your impressive krav maga fighting system in the future."

> —**Lt. Kevin Cowan**, Training Officer, New Jersey State Police,
> Executive Protection Bureau

"I would like to start by saying what an informative and eye-opening experience all of my team had during the seminar you and your team delivered in Portsmouth (UK) back in July 2013. The magnitude of knowledge combined with your relentless approach to adapting techniques to create a workable solution fit for specific military purpose was commendable. However, what stood out most to my team in our reflection of the experience was the manner of its delivery, as at no stage did you sell the system as being the way or a better way; you simply provided realistic options that could be adapted to fit any requirement or scenario/environment. Royal Marines Close Combat (RM CC) will always look to evolve, as this is at the heart of commando business. To cross-pollinate further knowledge and experiences I and my team will look to maintain links wherever possible with you and your instructors, as I strongly believe this will benefit to both parties, as I know you already do with other elite units globally."

> —**Sgt. Ben Perkins**, RM CC UK Chief Instructor Trainer (IT),
> Commando Training Centre Royal Marines

"I can personally attest to how effective krav maga under David Kahn really works. Many people train krav maga on a regular basis, but never get to use it outside the gym setting or in a real-life situation like I have. As a former professional football player, a police officer for twenty-two years, and a SWAT team member for 12 years, I know the need for proper and consistent training. I have found that training with David Kahn is the best for the patrol and SWAT officer. My real-life experience occurred when having to take into custody a wanted person who was a real threat to my life and possibly to those living in his area. One of my fellow officers who had just trained with David got to witness first hand the knowledge and training that David has taught the law enforcement community when I had to use krav maga to take the violent individual into custody. As a police officer studying krav maga under David Kahn it has change my life both mentally and physically. I have a confidence and knowledge in krav maga that I can only get from David!"

—Officer Al "Poodie" Carson

Of all the training I have put myself through for the last several years, nothing could have prepared me for the experience in Mexico City this evening. I am currently here on a business trip and was walking from the IBM office to my hotel (only ten minutes away) with two of my colleagues from the States. Some guy comes out of nowhere and started speaking Spanish in a threatening tone. I didn't know what he was saying, but he pulled out a gun and pointed it at all of us, moving it around (in broad daylight). All three of us froze up. One of my colleagues started trying to speak Spanish, saying sorry, no problem. I charged in and grabbed the gun followed by the standard disarm: redirected it to the ground, punched him so bloody hard in the face whilst keeping the gun pointed away, and pulled the gun out. He fell to the ground . . . I wanted to send you this note, because I know that krav maga and what I have learnt from you saved me.

—Anuj Batra, krav maga student

I have had the pleasure, opportunity, and advantage the last decade to train with the United States chief instructor of the Israeli Krav Maga Association, David Kahn. I first met David when I was assigned to the New Jersey State Police Training Academy in Sea Girt, New Jersey, as the lead defensive tactics instructor. I had been tasked by the commandant to research, evaluate, assess, and conduct a "best practices" for the NJSP defensive tactics program regarding duties of a NJSP trooper.

After researching federal, state, and local agencies' defensive tactics standards, training, and requirements, it was apparent that no uniform standard existed. However, it was obvious the Israeli Krav Maga Association met and exceeded any and all needs of the NJSP as well as the law enforcement community. I invited and met with David and his staff, as well as Haim Gidon, grandmaster for the Israeli Krav Maga Association based in Israel. After initially training with David it was clear that IKMA curriculum and best practices exceeded any national defensive tactics standards.

I noted that not all krav maga is the same and made the recommendation. I was granted permission by the commandant to move forward to formally bring in David Kahn. As a result,

Israeli krav maga was officially implemented into NJSP Academy recruit training, advanced, and in-service member training. David personally trained me, along with self-defense instructors Tpr. M. Oehlmann, Tpr. Rayhon, and Tpr. R. Roberts. David also trained the NJSP TEAMS (SWAT) and Executive Protection Unit (EPU). The IKMA provided us with the mind-set and physical skills a law enforcement officer will need to survive a situation and win. Several federal agencies have also brought David in to their academies to provide training for their instructors as well.

Training in IKM prepared members of the NJSP to react decisively, instinctively, and with speed and economy of motion, while combining a simultaneous defense and aggressive, objectively reasonable response that can be performed under pressure, thwarting any attack. IKM provided members with subduing techniques to safely and effectively direct, ease, place, restrain, and control an adversary onto the ground, thus limiting liability and enabling the trooper a smooth transition into a handcuffing procedure. IKM focused on legally acceptable anatomical targets, allowing female and male troopers alike to overcome and neutralize a stronger adversary while also complying with an objectively reasonable use-of-force standard. The integration of IKM provided members with a seamless transition from defensive and close-quarters combat tactics to firearms utilizing force options.

I highly recommend and believe that training with David Kahn (IKMA) should be implemented into all law enforcement agencies' firearms and defensive tactics programs. IKM is essential and critical to the responsibilities and job performance of law enforcement members and agencies.

> —**Mickie W. McComb (ret.)**, New Jersey State Police, Assistant unit head, Firearms and Self-Defense Training Unit; lead defensive tactics instructor and use of force instructor, Training Bureau, Sea Girt, New Jersey, Expert witness, excessive use of force: www.mickiemccombexpertwitnessuseofforce .com, The TASA Group—Technical Advisory Service for Attorneys: Expert witness, excessive use of force

David Kahn is a true professional. He is extremely knowledgeable yet humble. David is an outstanding author and instructor. I have known and worked with David for over fifteen years. This book will provide readers an opportunity to learn from one of the best Israeli krav maga instructors at their leisure. The techniques in this book are proven and effective. If practiced regularly and perfected, the techniques will become instinctive and will be effective. This book is the opportunity for you to better prepare yourself for encounters on the street or anywhere else. Now is the time to begin. Protect yourself, your comrades, and your family.

> —**Paul M. Miller**, retired captain, New Jersey State Police, academy instructor, TEAMS unit member

KRAV MAGA
PROFESSIONAL TACTICS

BECAUSE NOT ALL KRAV MAGA IS THE SAME™ . . .
"IMITATION IS THE SINCEREST FORM OF FLATTERY."
—Charles Caleb Colton

KRAV MAGA

PROFESSIONAL TACTICS

DAVID KAHN

THE CONTACT COMBAT SYSTEM OF THE ISRAEL DEFENSE FORCES

YMAA Publication Center
Wolfeboro, N.H., USA

YMAA Publication Center, Inc.
Main Office:
PO Box 480
Wolfeboro, New Hampshire, 03894
1-800-669-8892 • info@ymaa.com • www.ymaa.com

ISBN: 9781594393556 (print) • ISBN: 9781594393563 (ebook)

First edition. Copyright © 2016 by David Kahn
Edited by T. G. LaFredo
Copyedit by Doran Hunter
Cover design by Axie Breen
Photos by Mimi Rowland and Rinaldo Rossi unless noted otherwise

10 9 8 7 6 5 4 3 2 1

Publisher's Cataloging in Publication

Names: Kahn, David, 1972– author.
Title: Krav maga professional tactics : the contact combat system of the Israel Defense Forces / David Kahn.
Description: First edition. | Wolfeboro, N.H. : YMAA Publication Center, [2016] | Includes bibliographical
    references and index. | Contents: Civilian, law enforcement, and military krav maga training—Defending
    the most common upper-body and lower-body attacks, throws, and counterthrows—Clinches, choke and
    takedown defenses, escorts, and ground survival—Impact-weapon combatives and defenses—Firearm cold
    combatives—Defending edged weapons: open handed and when your handgun is inoperable—Multiple
    assailants—Firearm defenses—Firearm retention and professional kravist weapon-defense drills—Use
    of force.
Identifiers: ISBN: 978-1-59439-355-6 (print) | 978-1-59439-356-3 (ebook) | LCCN: 2016933951
Subjects: LCSH: Krav maga. | Krav maga—Training. | Self-defense. | Self-defense—Training. |
    Hand-to-hand fighting. | Hand-to-hand fighting—Training. | Martial arts—Training. |
    BISAC: SPORTS & RECREATION / Martial Arts & Self-Defense.
Classification: LCC: GV1111 .K25 2016 | DDC: 796.81—dc23

For Claire, Benjamin, and Leo
In Loving Memory of Helen Brener Smith and Master Lowell Slaven

The Book of Psalms, chapter 144:1

לדוד ברוך ה׳ צורי המלמד ידי
לקרב אצבעותי למלחמה

"A Psalm of David. Blessed be the LORD, my rock,
Who trains my hands for battle,
And my fingers for war."

Contents

Foreword: The Warrior Mind-Set

Having the physical and mental capability to negate a threat to your life and the lives of loved ones must be sharpened through tough, realistic training. Many people study and hone their combat mind-set skills. Much of this is done through the mental preparation for combat or a violent encounter. While mental preparation is highly important, one must hone the physical attributes to survive a violent altercation of any kind. Both of these subjects are imperative when a threat enters your OODA loop—that is, the decision-making cycle in which you observe, orient, decide, and act.

The techniques taught to me by Mr. Kahn, many of which are illustrated in this book, are highly efficient, effective, and practical. *These* techniques along with rigorous mental preparation can give you the combat mind-set and skills needed to survive a violent altercation. These techniques are a force multiplier to anyone's martial arts arsenal. As a military professional and a subject-matter expert in military hand-to-hand combat, it is my opinion that he is an unparalleled teacher and mentor. I would recommend his training to anyone. I recommend *Krav Maga Professional Tactics* by Mr. David Kahn to anyone serious about self-defense or lifesaving tactics.

—MSgt. (ret.) Ronald E. Jacobs

Ron Jacobs is the former chief instructor of the Marine Corps Martial Arts Program. His other martial arts credentials include the following:
Black belt, krav maga
Black belt, Japanese ju-jitsu
Kru (master instructor), muay Thai
Brown belt, Brazilian jiu-jitsu

Acknowledgements

I am indebted to Grandmaster Haim Gidon for instilling in me the self-defense fighting style of krav maga at its highest and most evolved level. As the head of the Israeli krav maga system and president of the Israeli Krav Maga Association (IKMA) Gidon System, Haim continues to develop and improve the krav maga system on a daily basis. With the blessing of Imi Lichtenfeld (the late founder of krav maga). Haim, along with the most capable assistance and expert insight from his sons (Albert, Ohad, and Noam) and other senior IKMA instructors represent the vanguard of krav maga development. I am also grateful to instructors Yoav Krayn, Yigal Arbiv and Steve Moishe. Haim emphasizes that the krav maga we teach must work against determined and concerted resistance; against someone who knows how to attack. or as Charles Caleb Colton summarized, "Imitation is the sincerest form of flattery." I can only hope that I can adequately represent Haim's unparalleled krav maga mastery.

I give special thanks to black-belt instructor Rinaldo Rossi for being both in front and behind the lens, along with Chris Eckel and Don Melnick for their unparalleled instructional support. Rinaldo is truly one of the world's foremost krav maga instructors and black-belt practitioners. This book would not exist without his dedication, patience, and generosity along with the help of Don and Chris. Instructor Mimi Rowland performed a nearly miraculous feat in helping to organize the many photos in addition to her creativity in shooting them. Thank you, Mimi.

It is an honor and privilege to work with my great friend Major HC "Sparky" Bollinger, ret. I first met Sparky at Camp Lejeune, North Carolina, through an introduction by our mutual friend Captain Frank Small, ret. Frank invited us to teach select marines at Camp Lejeune and persuaded Sparky, fresh off a flight from the Helmand Province after his second tour of duty, to attend the training. I knew right away that Sparky was a pro when it came to martial arts training. We were very appreciative of Sparky's acceptance and recognition that our krav maga "was good to go." A great friendship developed, as well as an atmosphere of mutual learning. Sparky holds a fifth-degree black belt in combat jujitsu and sits on the board of the United States Judo Association. He is a true comrade.

I am deeply grateful also to my close friend and business partner Captain Frank Small (ret.) and to his wonderful wife, Dana. Frank made it possible for us to work with the United States military. He quickly grasped the most important criterion for success in professional training: only what works. With this mind-set, he has paved the way for us to work with some of the finest professional warriors in America, including M.Sgt. Ronald E. Jacobs, chief instructor for the United States Marine Corps Martial Arts Program. Ron holds a sixth-degree black belt in MCMAP along with high-ranking belts in numerous other martial arts systems, including a black belt in Israeli krav maga. It is an honor and privilege to work with Ron, who was gracious enough to pose in several of the photo series presented in this book. He is a consummate professional and a great friend.

I am grateful to Navy instructors R., J., N., J., and S. for their nonpareil professional insights, hospitality, and most, importantly, for what they do.

Sgt. Major Nir Maman, res., former LOTAR lead counterterror instructor, krav maga instructor, and IDF Infantry and Paratroopers Ground Forces Command Soldier of the Year, 2009, has provided great support, professional insights, and specialized training expertise as only he can. Nir has improved the Israeli krav maga system immeasurably with his unique professional insights. Nir is also one of my greatest friends.

I am grateful to my other Israeli krav maga instructors and close friends. Aldema Tzrinksky is a great friend who has provided immeasurable support and counsel over many years. Many thanks to the Hauerstocks for their *sabra* hospitality in my biannual visits to Israel and my good friend Shira Orbas, now one of the best in the security "business," along with her wonderful family. I offer special thanks to Master Kobi Lichtenstein and his organization for their hospitality.

Thank you to the IKMA board of directors and all IKMA members, who continue to welcome and train with me over the years. Once again, this book would not be possible without the expert training, support, and inspiration of krav maga's backbone: the IKMA (www.kravmagaisraeli.com).

The same is true of senior krav maga instructors Rick Blitstein and Alan Feldman, who are support strongholds and knowledge reservoirs. Their collective sagacity improves me as an instructor. Our good friend in Poland, Kris Sawicki, keeps the IKMA at the forefront in Europe. A special thanks to USJA master instructor Lowel Slaven for his considerable vote of confidence and professional interest. I am grateful to all our students at our Israeli Krav Maga United States Training Centers (www.israelikrav.com).

I am indebted to many other friends, supporters, and my network of fellow instructors in the krav maga world: Chris Eckel, Jeff Gorman, Frank Colluci, Mike Delahanty, David Ordini, Alec Goenner, David Gollin, George Foster, Jason Bleitstein, Joe Tucker, David Rahn, Chris Morrison, Al Ackerman, Joe Drew, Jose Anaya, Kelly Arlinghaus, Mimi Rowland, Mike McElvin, and Paul Karleen, along with all those instructors in the pipeline.

Thanks to A. B. Duki and Marc of the Residence Beach Hotel (www.zyvotels.com) for hosting our biannual training stays in Netanya. A. J. Yolofsky and Enrique Prado deserve thanks for their public support and efforts. I am also grateful to Kim and Oliver Pimley for their dedication and to Art Co for his support and for explaining the nuances of Philippine edged-weapons tactics. The Tenenbaums and Goldbergs remain pillars of my life and *mishpachat*. I'd like to give special thanks to the family of James Gandolfini and John Mayer for their trust and backing. I also extend my thanks to Justin Kingson and the late Bill Kingson.

A special thanks on both a personal and professional level to all of our friends and supporters in the law enforcement community, including Lt. Miller, ret.; Sgt. McComb, ret.; Sgt. Klem; Sgt. Oehlmann; Sgt. Rayhon; Maj. Ponenti; Lt. DeMaise; Lt. Wolf; Lt. Cowan; Sgt. Boland; Lt. Capriglione; Lt. Peins; Officer Vaval; Capt. Crowe; Officer Vacirca; Capt. Maimone, ret.; Lt. Cowan; Capt. Savalli, ret.; Associate Director Harrison; Chief Lazzarotti; Director Paglione; Investigators Smith and Gioscio; Officer Tucker; Officer Hanafee; Lt. Colon; Sgt. Hayden; Officer Johnson; Special Agent-in-Charge Hammond; Special Agents Schroeder and Belle; Special Agents Love, Clark, Nowazcek, and Crowe; Chief Sutter, Lt. Currier, and my entire hometown Princeton Police Department, along with the many other law enforcement professionals with whom we have the honor of working.

I would like to thank the following United States Marine Corps personnel: Lt. Col. Joseph Shusko, ret.; GySgt. Gokey, ret.; MGySgt. Urso, ret.; Sgts. Ladler, Parker, and Allen; Lt. Col. "Tonto" Ardese; SSgt. Jensen; Cpl. Lackland; and SSgt. Kropelwicki. Thanks also to Sgt. Ben Perkins of the Royal Marines, along with 1st Sgt. Johnson and Maj. Haigh of the United States Air Force for their support. I must not fail to mention all of our fighting men and women of the United States military and Israel Defense Forces for safeguarding our freedom.

Security expert Steven Hartov, one of my favorite authors and good friends, deserves much gratitude for his personal and professional support. I am grateful to Drs. Steven Gecha, Stephen Hunt, and Bruce Rose, as well as PTs Lindsey Balint and Jeff Manheimer for continuing to hold me together. Thanks to Jerry Palmieri for his conditioning advice along with George Samuelson and "Doc" Mark Cheng.

My family is always a buttress and the wellspring of support, especially my wife Claire, mother Anne, stepfather Ed, and father Alfred, for the growth of krav maga training and all the effort that has gone into our expansion. My business partners are true brothers to me, embodying the greatest dedication, entrepreneurial spirit, work ethic, and loyalty. I trust Benjamin and Leo will be the next generation of kravists—and be more accomplished than their daddy.

I am especially grateful to my publisher David Ripianzi for recognizing the need for a comprehensive krav maga book featuring many professional tactics, strategies, and insights of the Israeli fighting method. David has also helped me in innumerable ways to improve as an author, video producer, and entrepreneur. Tim Comrie, Doran Hunter, and T. G. LaFredo each warrant deep thanks as well for each expert's respective role in shaping this book. YMAA Publication Center is a credit to the profession, and I am honored to work with such a great group of professional people.

Introduction

We are proud to present *Krav Maga Professional Tactics*. We thank the many readers and krav maga enthusiasts who contacted us about the next book of the line. Here, you will learn more about the proven core, and in some cases, advanced combative and weapon tactics of the Israel Defense Forces developed first by Imi Lichtenfeld and refined by Grandmaster Haim Gidon. Sgt. Maj. Nir Maman, res., has also made significant contributions to the Israeli krav maga system. The tactics and strategies represented in this book have established their efficacy in defeating aggression over the last seven decades.

I have selected many techniques from the top levels of krav maga. There are several tactics we elected not to include for security considerations in the public interest. Obviously, these omitted offensive and third-party protection tactics are singularly suited for training vetted personnel. I am confident this omission does not detract from the principles and tactics detailed in this book.

Krav maga's popularity in professional law enforcement, military, and security circles is, in large part, attributable to its practicality, simplicity, quick retention, easy learning curve, and brutal effectiveness. We train federal, state, and local law enforcement agencies along with all four branches of the US military in the method. We have also trained foreign military branches and private security contractors.

I would like to reiterate a quick anecdote from *Krav Maga Weapon Defenses* (YMAA, 2012). Over the years we have had several skeptical highly skilled operators take our courses to disprove Israeli krav maga's professional applications and effectiveness. As far as we are aware, none of these warriors came away unimpressed with krav maga. Some were more than impressed and asked to be put on our mailing list for all future courses.

We are firmly rooted to the precept that good tactical minds think alike. Our goal is not to replace whatever knowledge these seasoned personnel have but rather to augment their capabilities, to add additional arrows to the proverbial quiver. What is paramount is that we do not approach our specific krav maga training as an exercise program or fad. The tactics and strategies we teach are designed by and for hard-core, no-nonsense, tactically minded professionals, along with civilians who are serious about safety training. *Not all krav maga is the same.* For those who convert these tactics and strategies for their own use without attribution, you know who you are. We know who you are.

The Professional Level

The Israeli krav maga self-defense system is world renowned for its brutal efficiency. The system's continuing evolution is grounded in street- and battle-proven tactics. If a tactic should fail, the system either removes it or modifies it. This effectiveness is built on a few core tenets and simple building blocks. Krav maga's street and battlefield survival defenses were developed for a modern army, the Israel Defense Force (IDF), as its official self-defense and close-quarters combat system. Modern armies, law enforcement agencies, and security forces need a hand-to-hand combat system based on simplicity, adaptability, practicality, and most important, defensive, instinctive movements. These professionals need a system that can be readily honed. Krav maga fits the bill.

Krav maga is often translated as "contact combat." The meaning here is significant. Combat is a life-and-death battle devoid of rules. This is the fundamental military under-pinning of the krav maga system's methods and philosophy. It also takes into account limitations that may be imposed on the defender's movements and flexibility due to equip-ment and weight loads, such as a duty belt, bulletproof vest, flak jacket, Kevlar helmet, or backpack. What a flexible, unencumbered mixed martial arts fighter wearing shorts may be able to accomplish in a ring is often a far cry from what a fully equipped operator or, equally important, average person may be able to accomplish in a combat zone or on the street, respectively.

In this book we continue to develop a self-defense fighting arsenal based on the green, blue, brown, and advanced-level black-belt techniques of Israeli krav maga. The techniques represented here focus on the most common violent scenarios law enforcement, security, and military personnel typically face—but civilians, on occasion, also find themselves in these dangerous encounters. These techniques derive from my translation of the Israeli Krav Maga Association (IKMA) technique guidelines. The expert insights of Sgt. Maj. Nir Maman, res., are also woven into the tactics.

The IKMA is the governing body for Israeli krav maga recognized by the Israeli government and headed by Grandmaster Haim Gidon. Haim Gidon received his eighth dan (black belt) ranking on June 5, 1996, when krav maga founder Imi Lichtenfeld also declared that ninth and tenth dans (red belt) were to come. Thus, Haim Gidon, after Imi's passing in 1998, became the highest-ranking krav maga instructor in the world, following in Imi's hallowed footsteps.

Haim introduced several key weapons technique modifications and improvements— all formally approved by krav maga founder Imi Lichtenfeld. While improving the system daily, Haim follows Imi's fundamental premise that krav maga must work for everyone, even against the most skilled adversaries—professionals. Constant enhance-ment, evolution, and adaptability make krav maga a most formidable fighting method. Its hallmark and genius is to teach anyone to successfully defend against deadly weapon attacks.

Krav maga's defensive philosophy is never to do more than necessary, but to react instinctively with violence of action involving speed, economy of motion, and the appro-priate measure of force. The basic principle is to do whatever is practical to deliver a defender from harm's way. Instinctive trained reaction is paramount. One is taught to strike instinctively at the human anatomy's vulnerabilities. The practitioner relies on being proactive, rather than reactive, as soon as possible.

The training attempts to place you in the most realistic pressure scenarios. The bottom line is to present trained instinctive solutions to defeat any threat in the most effective way possible. This includes the decisive use of lethal force when warranted. Krav maga uses the same building blocks from the simplest defenses to the most advanced techniques, including empty-handed defenses and disarming techniques against bladed weapons, firearms, and even a microexplosive—as you will soon learn.

The system stresses several adaptable core tactics, and its application is flexible in line with its modern combat evolution. Real-life encounters account for modification, revision, and the addition of new techniques. While krav maga weapons defenses are specific, their application must be adaptable to accommodate the unpredictability of a violent confrontation. Stated another way, we apply general principles but customize them to suit the needs of a given violent situation. Most important, krav maga emphasizes that there are no rules in a deadly encounter. Do whatever is necessary to overcome the threat in a life-or-death situation and *survive*.

Core tenets of each defense involve deflection-redirections, evasive footwork, and upper-body movements combined with simultaneous or near-simultaneous counter-attacks to overwhelm the assailant. Importantly, the defensive tactics are designed for multiple-assailant encounters to protect the defender, incapacitate the assailant(s), and, when necessary, commandeer the assailant's weapon for the defender's use. Krav maga instills an *attack-the-assailant mind-set*, providing the defender with an all-important preemption capability prior to a weapon's active deployment. The defender's goal is to take away the assailant's freedom of action. Of course, recognition of the warning signs of impending violence allows a defender to thwart an attack at its inception.

Israeli krav maga's stellar reputation is built on the following four pillars:

1. It emphasizes defending against any manner of attack (unarmed or armed).
2. It relies on instinctive body movements, which are honed, easily learned, retained, and performed under stress.
3. The techniques are based on building blocks that, when combined, allow the defender to prevail in life-threatening situations.
4. Defenders react with speed, economy of motion, and the appropriate measure of force.

Three Reaction-Proaction Levels

Level I: Common-sense reactions. At the common-sense novice level, your reactions to violence are still somewhat conscious. You still deliberate over your reactions, which have not yet become instinctive. Conditioned reflexive responses are not yet a part of the novice's arsenal. Movements are not yet fluid. A counterattack is a catch-up *reaction* to attack or defensive response, not an *action* to thwart an incipient attack.

Level II: Proficient reactions. You reach this level when your subconscious assumes control and you *react* as the attack is initiated. You now respond instinctively to any threat and quickly assume control over the situation. By recognizing the attack or preparatory movements, you instinctively comprehend the threat descending on you. When confronted with danger, you automatically respond as you have practiced or visualized. You are approaching a high level of proficiency.

Level III: Instantaneous trained reactions. This expert-level *kravist* takes the initiative through preemptive action. Initiative and prescribed controlled movement take over the millisecond you recognize the threat. This allows you to seamlessly execute your thwarting action. In other words, you attack the assailant. You instantaneously recall a scenario you have mentally stored through action, practice, or visualization and explode into preemptive action without the slightest hesitation. The advanced or expert level-III kravist will recognize that same attack before the assailant can initiate.

Fight Timing

Essential to a successful defense is correct fight timing: using the appropriate tactic at the correct time. Preemption and fight timing are a fusion of instinct with simultaneous decision-making. You have the choice to either preempt an opponent's attack by initiating your own attack or respond to the opponent's attack, countertargeting a physical vulnerability the opponent exposes. In other words, even when skilled, an opponent when attacking leaves himself briefly open for counterattack. For example, as the opponent delivers a straight punch, he shifts his weight forward, offering you the opportunity to deliver a side kick to damage the knee of his lead leg. Fight timing is harnessing instinctive body movements while seizing or creating opportunities to defend both effectively and logically.

Fight timing, alternatively defined, is the defender's ability to capitalize on a window of opportunity offered by the adversary, or to create an opportunity to end the confrontation using whatever tactics come instinctively. Timing must be developed and sharpened with realistic training—always krav maga's objective. While speed is not timing, speed can deliver a decisive advantage when the defender acts more quickly than the assailant. As emphasized throughout this book, krav maga relies on economy of motion to eliminate wasted movement, which, in turn, improves speed.

The Best Use of This Book

This book is designed for security-conscious civilians, law enforcement officers, military personnel, and security professionals alike who wish to improve their chances of surviving an armed attack and prevailing without serious injury. The best use of this book is to practice each technique as presented. You'll find that each technique either builds upon a previous technique or compliments a technique presented later.

Again, the Israeli krav maga system relies on a few core self-defense tactics adaptable to most violent encounters. No book is a substitute for hands-on learning with a qualified Israeli krav maga expert instructor, but our goal is to impart some of the more important principles and core tactics to hone one's self-defense skills in the specific situations we cover and, by extension, other similar situations. Be sure to thoroughly vet any instructor with whom you should decide to train because *not all krav maga is the same.*

CHAPTER 1
Civilian, Law Enforcement, and Military Krav Maga Training

Responsible people pursue krav maga training as a shield against violence, *not as a weapon to orchestrate violence*. Krav maga training for civilians, law enforcement, and military personnel all share the same principle: to deliver oneself from harm's way. Importantly, the "ending" or end goal is different. The exception is when any category of defender faces a situation involving deadly force. The following table summarizes the engagement strategies with the key end-goal differentiations for civilians, law enforcement, and military:

Civilian:	Law enforcement:	Military:
• disrupt	• disrupt	• disrupt
• incapacitate as necessary	• incapacitate	• incapacitate or maim
• disengage; call police	• subjugate and control or, if necessary, terminate	• terminate

As noted, the core tenets and building blocks of Israeli krav maga are taught to civilians, law enforcement, and military personnel alike. The crucial difference, again, is the "finish." Regardless of one's professional standing or state-granted immunity, if you are faced with a life-threatening attack, you are generally justified in using lethal counterforce. For civilians or law enforcement, three elements must be present to warrant the use of counterforce: an assailant must have the (1) intent, (2) means, and (3) capability to cause bodily harm.

In a legal use-of-force analysis, civilians may use counterforce commensurate with the amount of force used on them. (Hence the term counterforce.) For law enforcement, however, most jurisdictions allow an officer or agent to escalate the use of counterforce one level higher. When an arrest must be made, law enforcement's goal is to use "objectively reasonable" force in taking a suspect into custody (*Graham v. Connor* 490 U.S. 386). When force is required, the goal remains the same while safeguarding both the officer and the

1

suspect. A deadly force encounter is just that: officers are facing down a perpetrator intent on severely injuring them or a third party.

My good friend, Sergeant First Class Mick McComb, ret., was kind enough to contribute on this matter (see appendix). Mick served twenty-five years with the New Jersey State Police. For ten years he was assigned to the NJSP Training Bureau. He is currently a federal court-accepted use-of-force expert and Israeli krav maga instructor.

For military personnel, krav maga focuses on lethal-force applications. These include the optimum offensive use of weaponry. Firearm or "hot weapon" lethal tactics, impact and edged-weapon lethal tactics, and techniques using all of your personal weapons—your limbs, head, teeth (if necessary)—are essential to professional krav maga training. Krav maga employs specific methods to strangle an enemy combatant or sever his spinal cord. We do not publish these tactics for public consumption.

> **There is a distinct difference between law enforcement and military krav maga training.** Not everyone understands or honors this important separation. For example, when training military police, we successfully tackle both spheres by combining elements where applicable and separating the law enforcement the military's respective end goals. It is vitally important that readers understand their end goal and the force the state empowers them to use. An unfortunate common mistake is to substitute law enforcement techniques for military techniques. To be sure, they can overlap, but military training, when taught properly, focuses on terminating an enemy combatant.

The Professional Kravist Mind-Set When Facing a Deadly Attack

Krav maga training focuses on the realistic and brutal nature of both self-defense and hand-to-hand combat. Targeting an opponent's vital and structural anatomy is essential to one's counterattack tactics and strategy. Breaking an opponent's anatomic functionality is central to hand-to-hand combat or defensive tactics in a deadly force encounter.

As is the goal with any reality-based training, you'll learn to avoid freezing under the stress and pressure of a violent encounter. You'll learn how to harness an instinctive and instantaneous trained reaction without thinking. You'll defend yourself from a visceral level—however you can. The goal is to react instantaneously, without thinking.

Training prepares you for any eventuality, so when you find yourself in a dangerous position, you will know you've been there and done that. What follows is an autonomic response. The techniques become not second nature, but first nature. The goal is that you never waiver or contemplate the life-threatening situation. Let your training hijack the circumstances. The optimal outcome is to neutralize the threat at its very inception.

To prepare a professional to face a potential deadly force street encounter or the realities of a modern-day battlefield, krav maga's training tactics include defending against full-force multiple attacks with facsimile impact and edged weapons. At the same time, we practice defending against firearm threats using Simunitions® to simulate firearm discharges. Note: always wear protective equipment in full-on training, including eye protection when working with facsimile weapons. Under strictly controlled conditions, we also allow trainees to secure a live firearm to discharge it down range to prove the defense will work.

There are six different levels of awareness in Israeli krav maga:

−5	−4	−3	−2	−1	0
Unaware	Semi-aware	Aware	Cautious	Alert	Prepared

Psychological Aspects of Violent Conflict

Violent conflict produces severe stress on the human mind, slowing down the cognitive process. Instincts will always dominate over cognitive response under stress. The limbic or primitive part of your brain ("unconscious mind") narrows the gap between reaction and action on the action-reaction power curve and cannot be cognitively controlled. The action-reaction power curve suggests that an action will generally beat a reaction, as the defender must "catch up" to counter the attack. Reducing the reaction time from recognition to action is vital in a defensive violent encounter.

The neocortex ("conscious mind") section of the brain is chiefly responsible for higher cognition and analysis. Paradoxically, the limbic and neocortical systems can be in competition or at odds regarding self-defense. The limbic system relies on the body's natural self-preservation actions, while the neocortex may try to make logical sense of an action or event. This is what causes us to freeze. When under physical duress, a person may have difficulty thinking clearly because his cognitive abilities are being suppressed by the limbic brain, which has asserted control over all cerebral functions.

Hormone levels (including cortisol), when affected by high stress, impair memory. Hence we see the importance of an instinctive or conditioned self-defense response. Instinctive (re)action harnesses adrenaline. As a result, the mind reverts to three processes: freeze, flight, or fight. If freezing is not the optimum response, the limbic brain orders flight or escape. If flight is impossible, the limbic brain's final mandate is to fight by converting fear into fury to physically confront a threat. Therefore, the self-defense and close-quarters battle (CQB) process may be understood using the following four-part process:

1. Threat recognition
2. Situation analysis
3. Choice of action
4. Action or inaction

Security professionals know well to accept the possibility of violence under any circumstances. Maintaining an overall strategy to take away your opponent's ability to harm you is paramount. If your actions require a forceful and debilitating physical response, krav maga will provide it. Remember, though, the intensity of your response will escalate to meet the threat.

Violent Conflict's Mental and Physical Stress Manifestations

It is well known that stress, when triggered in a potentially violent situation, protects the body. Mental and physical stress can produce shock. When confronting a life-threatening situation, shock can be more problematic then fear. Uncontrolled shock causes the body's homeostasis to cease, and it can no longer compensate for injuries. The body begins a shutdown procedure, which beyond a certain point becomes irreversible.

Through training, krav maga's goal is to embed in your subconscious with preparation and conditioning of the highest order. The key is to transition immediately from surprise to an assault mind-set. One must be aware of the following:

- Tunnel vision: under extreme stress, to increase blood and oxygen delivery to the eyes, one's attention may be focused primarily on the greatest threat, resulting in a temporary loss of peripheral vision.

- Auditory exclusion: one's vision takes over as the primary sense, diminishing one's hearing.

- Compression of time and space: time and space will become muddled with added difficulty in judging the interrelationship of speed and distance. Movements may appear in slow motion.

Before any violent encounter, regardless of the specific circumstances, you must adopt a winner-take-all mind-set under any and all circumstances—a no-lose, locked-on attitude. While you cannot underestimate the assailant's abilities, the assailant's abilities, paradoxically, are irrelevant—provided your intent and determination surpass the assailant's. That must be your mind-set. With superior determination combined with a honed krav maga skill set, you will have the decisive advantage. You will win. You will survive.

To help make krav maga first nature, one must also train mentally to defeat *any* threat, to know one's training and determination will prevail regardless of who or what may confront the defender. Mental assurance, combined with physical preparedness, provides a decisive advantage to triumph in a violent encounter. Of course, there is a fine distinction between confidence and overconfidence. Do not mistake the latter for the former. In short, believe your training will unleash your own violence of action that will carry the day regardless of an adversary's capabilities.

Krav Maga's Training Philosophy

Krav maga is designed around a few core tactics to counter a myriad of attacks. Defenders get tools for their toolboxes along with a general blueprint for how to use them. Imi's goal was survival in any defensible situation. While there are no set solutions for ending an armed confrontation, there are preferred methods using violence of action combined with *retzev*, or "continuous combat motion." A few mastered techniques go a long way and are highly effective against both unarmed and armed threats and attacks. The defender learns how to protect his vital points and organs. Equally important, the defender perfects how to debilitate an adversary through anatomical targeting.

Retzev teaches the defender to move instinctively in combat motion without *thinking* about the next logical move. In short, the defender launches a seamless, overwhelming counterattack using strikes, takedowns, throws, joint locks, chokes, or other offensive actions combined with evasive action. Retzev, armed or unarmed, is quick and decisive movement merging all aspects of one's krav maga training. Defensive movements transition automatically into offensive movements to neutralize the attack, leaving an adversary little or no time to react.

Retzev may be compared to a professional law enforcement or military assault. Professional military and law enforcement personnel use overwhelming violence of action and a preponderance of firepower. Criminals try to do the same. The predatory assault mind-set is ruthless and controlled; it detaches the target from human to either a target resource or target threat. Therefore, if attacked, the kravist must—within the boundaries of the law—become the most viscerally violent person present, capable of defeating any threat.

Combined with simultaneous defense and attack, retzev is a seamless, decisive, and overwhelming counterattack, forming the backbone of the Israeli fighting system. When defending against weapons, retzev is modified ("modified weapons retzev") because the nearside arm often controls the assailant's weapon or weapon arm. Krav maga uses retzev to overwhelm an assailant to complete the defense. It combines upper- and lower-body combatives, locks, chokes, throws, takedowns, and weapons interchangeably without pause.

From a professional's standpoint, violence is paradoxically both unpredictable and predictable, due to one's prior experience and training. There is one certainty regarding violence: there are none. Even with the best training, you may find yourself in a "negative five" position—which is to say initially unprepared for the fight of your life. An assailant, seeking every advantage, will try to catch you off guard.

Field experience, proper training, or both can trigger an automatic fighting response. Realistic training improves reaction capability by allowing an immediate assessment of a violent situation and triggering a corresponding stress-simulated reaction. An attack launched by surprise can force you to react from an unprepared state. Therefore, a self-defense reaction must be instinctive and reflexive. Training ingrains the appropriate responses; whether the threat comes from an edged weapon or gun, you will already know how to react. Training puts honed instinct in control.

Visceral Counterviolence

A kravist's violent intent governs his violence of action. True self-defense or counterviolence focuses not simply on survival but rather on how to optimally injure, cripple, maim, and—if necessary and justified—kill. If you begin with the intent to injure and neutralize your opponent, a trained paroxysm of counterviolence is more likely to favorably conclude the situation. Use the closest weapon to attack the closest target. Your goal is to achieve traumatic injury in the shortest time, using the most opportune route. Target the opponent's vulnerable anatomy, damage that anatomy, continue to damage it, and capitalize on debilitating him to move on to the next anatomical target as necessary. Inflicting injury obviously affords the opportunity to impose more injury. For example, delivering a debilitating side kick to an adversary's knee usually immobilizes him, exposing him to your further onslaught. In short, a kravist's rapid infliction of successive damage, mutilation, and wounds epitomizes the optimum use of counterviolence.

Attack the Attacker: Anatomical Targeting

To stop an assailant, krav maga primarily targets the body's vital soft tissue, chiefly the groin, neck, and eyes. Other secondary targets include the kidneys, solar plexus, knees, liver, joints, fingers, nerve centers, and other smaller, fragile bones. The professional immediately recognizes that an assailant might also target these same targets and, accordingly, takes measures to protect his own vital anatomy. A protective posture or stance is integral to krav maga training. In addition, krav maga teaches you to disarm assailants and, if necessary, turn the weapon against them. The system differs from other systems that may rely primarily on targeting difficult-to-locate nerve centers.

Forging an awareness of your own personal weapons and an adversary's vulnerabilities is essential to fight strategy and tactics, especially when he is armed and you are not. There are no rules in a fight, particularly in the life-or-death struggle of combat. This lack of rules distinguishes the system from sport fighting.

Krav maga, initially developed as a military fighting discipline, employs lethal-force techniques. Lethal force may involve crushing the skull, cutting off an aggressor's oxygen supply or blood flow, severing the spine or major arteries, or stopping or penetrating the heart, along with several other slower-acting methods of inflicting trauma. Founder Imi Lichtenfeld was resolute that these techniques remain confined to military and professional security circles. While these techniques are integrated at the highest levels of the IKMA curriculum, trainees who are exposed to them are highly vetted.

A key to krav maga—especially for law enforcement, security, and military professionals, along with legally armed citizens—is understanding weapon deployment and the capabilities of different categories of weapons. Those categories include *personal* (hands, forearms, elbows, knees, shins, feet, and head), *cold* (impact and edged weapons, plus firearms used as impact weapons), and *hot* (firearms). Another key is making a seamless transition from one weapon type to another.

In both defending and attacking, recognizing the human anatomy's vulnerabilities is essential to fight strategy and tactics. The human body is amazingly resilient. Therefore, an adversary may only be stopped when his offensive capabilities are put out of commission by nonlethal concussive force, joint dislocations, bone breaks, or cutting off the blood supply to the brain, resulting in unconsciousness. If necessary, krav maga also employs chokes and "blood" chokes to render an adversary unconscious or worse.

From a professional standpoint, even when an attacker is shot with a large-caliber round, it is well documented that he or she may continue to fight. Therefore, the defender must not let down his guard or cease defensive actions until the threat is neutralized. Medical research in one study indicates that 64 percent of those who were shot and received wounds to the chest and abdomen continued to fight for more than five minutes after being wounded. Moreover, 36 percent of those who sustained wounds to the head and neck continued to function for more than five minutes, some still capable of continuing violent offensive actions.[1] These facts have been historically borne out when, in self-defense, Israeli security forces have shot terrorists who nevertheless continued to attack.

A wounded terrorist can continue an attack even when shot multiple times, and this was underscored during an attack in Jerusalem on October 13, 2015. A terrorist rammed his car into a number of civilians waiting at a bus stop. The terrorist exited his vehicle and continued his attack with a meat cleaver, killing an Israeli citizen. A security guard who witnessed the attack closed on the terrorist and shot the terrorist multiple times at close range. The terrorist continued to struggle and attempted to continue his attack nearly thirty seconds after being shot repeatedly at close range.

This type of terrorist attack with an edged weapon (and with firearms) is, unfortunately, a regular occurrence in Israel. The lessons learned remain the same when dealing with wounded attackers who will continue their deadly onslaught until physically shut down. Hence, the Israeli security forces have a standard operating procedure when neutralizing terrorists. Note: knowing when to cease fire is specific to every incident and not a clear cut or easy decision to make. The subject matter is not within the scope of this book (see footnote 1 for a insightful analysis and recommended reading).

---

[1] Law Enforcement Executive Forum, 2014, 14(2). Police Officer Reaction Time to Start and Stop Shooting: The Influence of Decision Making and Pattern Recognition by William J. Lewinski, William B. Hudson, Jennifer L Dyster-theft citing research from Adams et al., 2009; Levy & Rao, 1988; Newgard, 1992, Spitz, Petty, & Fisher, 1961.

With proper body positioning, an adversary on the ground can be pummeled severely while giving him little defensive recourse. Logically, in both standing and ground fights, it becomes difficult for an adversary to fight effectively if his hands or limbs are broken, and rendering an adversary unconscious quickly ends a fight. Every type of lock requires moving the joint against its natural articulation with breaking pressure. While we teach certain core arm dislocation positions, once you have an understanding of the biomechanics, you can apply the principles to many situations. This is especially important in the fluidity of a fight. Optimally, you will use the entire force and weight of your body to apply pressure against an adversary's joint. This is the key principle to joint locks. Remember that a joint lock, however decisive and quick, still ties you up momentarily, exposing you to a second adversary—or multiple adversaries—attacking you.

Remember, standing, clinched, or on the ground, krav maga is designed for everyone. A smaller opponent can defeat a larger, stronger, and perhaps more athletic opponent. A well-trained kravist will possess core training in all three combat phases. In a rapidly unfolding fighting chess match, the best way to defend against an offensive technique is to know the offensive technique. Knowing an array of techniques solidifies your ability at an advanced level.

Twenty-Four Vulnerable Targets

In krav maga, you learn to avoid hard skeletal bones such as the back of the head and rib cage, and focus your efforts on easy-to-strike soft tissues. Good targets include the following:

1. Temples
2. Eyes
3. Ears
4. Nose
5. Chin and jaw
6. Throat (specifically the windpipe)
7. Sides, back, and hollow of the neck
8. Base of the skull
9. Base of the neck
10. The spinal column
11. Clavicles
12. Fingers
13. Solar plexus
14. Elbows
15. Ribs
16. Liver
17. Spleen
18. Back and kidneys
19. Stomach
20. Testicles
21. Thighs
22. Knees
23. Ankles
24. Top of the foot

Pain may stop some assailants, but others have enormous pain thresholds. Therefore, an opponent may only be decisively stopped when his offensive capabilities are put out of commission by joint dislocations, bone breaks, or by cutting off the oxygen or blood supply to the brain, resulting in unconsciousness.

Injuring versus Hurting

Spinal reflexes govern the body's physical reaction to damage. While physically resilient, the human body is affected by structural injury in a somewhat predictable manner. Therefore, a kravist can generally predict how his counterattacks will affect the assailant's subsequent movements or capabilities. Strategically, inflicting a first-salvo injury against an adversary opens the door to unleash subsequent injurious counterattacks. As another example, when an attacker is hit in the face, usually his head will jolt backward, exposing his throat and neck to attack while also forcing his pelvis forward to expose his groin for further attack. As emphasized, the optimum way to end a violent conflict is to injure the opponent rapidly and repeatedly as necessary.

Deadly, concerted, one-on-one, up-close-and-personal violence usually lasts no more than a few seconds. Adopting a simple survival mind-set is inadequate; you must not get seriously injured or maimed. One usually does not cleanly win a violent hand-to-hand combat encounter. One survives it, subject to an injury scale. Krav maga, at its core, does not reflect "fighting" prowess so much as the ability to damage the adversary. In a fight, experienced combatants understand that specific defensive tactics rarely work or are applied. Rather, it is your offensive capabilities that are paramount. A well-timed, decisive preemptive attack creating anatomical damage, followed by additional combatives, usually prevails. In other words, the victor is whichever fighter first successfully exploits an anatomical vulnerability of his opponent with a well-placed debilitating combative and, then, continues to serially injure the opponent through retzev continuous combat motion.

Importantly, it is an ambush situation, or the negative five, where a specific defensive tactic designed to counter a particular threat or attack may be successfully employed. In other words, by necessity, the ambushed defensive party reacts first defensively and then, as soon as possible, transitions to the counterattack. Conversely, when engaged in mutual combat, offensive capabilities take priority and come to the fore. The one who first imposes a debilitating injury and then follows through with additional combatives is usually the one who prevails. An analogy might be a well-placed bullet from a semiautomatic weapon followed by that weapon's then going fully automatic to finish the threat. When facing a potential lethal encounter, every counterviolent act should focus on inflicting injury or damage to render the aggressor incapable of further aggression.

When there is no choice but to use counterviolence, a professional kravist is compelled to maim, cripple, or—provided the circumstances are legally justifiable—kill an assailant by, say, breaking bones, disabling ligaments, or destroying an eyeball. In short, and in an animalistic sense, inflicting terrible, debilitating wounds on an adversary—maiming an assailant—balances power in the kravist's favor.

It is axiomatic that the party who significantly damages the other party first usually prevails if he presses the counterattack home to neutralize the threat. Once again, there is no pity or humanity in visceral self-defense or hand-to-hand combat, *provided* the ends justify the means in the correct use of force. Survivors do not waver in believing they will impose their will on an aggressor to alter the outcome.

Legal Considerations

However and wherever krav maga self-defense might be used, it must be legally justifiable. For anyone acting outside of law enforcement or military duties, counterforce must be commensurate (including one level above) with the threat and meet an "objectively reasonable" standard for the given circumstances. Those employing self-defense will need to articulate why they had no choice when faced with a threat who demonstrated all of the following:

- Intent (stated or evident goal of harming you)
- Capability (prowess or tools to harm you)
- Opportunity (proximity)

If any of the above three criteria is absent or becomes absent—or if you could avoid the threat altogether—you are no longer acting in self-defense. While this book focuses on professional krav maga applications, they must always be used for the right reason—self-defense with the appropriate level of counterforce. The following table serves as a summary and reference for the Israeli krav maga system's philosophy, tactics, and strategy:

The Professional Krav Maga Four Pillars Tactical Grid©

Deliver simultaneous defense and attack.	Focus on vulnerable soft tissue and anatomy.
Combine your defense and offense into one complete strategy. Do whatever is necessary to overcome a dangerous threat.	Counterattack the vulnerable areas of your adversary's body, including the groin, eyes, and throat.
Act with retzev, or continuous combat motion.	Master a few instinctive tactics.
Move fast, continuously, seamlessly, and determinedly—when necessary, attacking with extreme prejudice, giving the assailant no time to react.	Learn a few core tactics and use them instinctively to prevail in a myriad of situations.

The Israeli Krav Maga Advantage

The key is your mind-set: to neutralize an opponent quickly and decisively. In fighting sports, the following tactics are generally banned: eye gouges, throat strikes, head butting, biting, hair pulling, clawing, pinching or twisting of the flesh, striking the spine and the back of the head, striking with the tip of the elbow, small-joint manipulation, kidney and liver strikes, clavicle strikes, kneeing or kicking the head of an opponent on the ground, and slamming an opponent to the ground on his head. These are exactly the combined core tactics krav maga emphasizes.

Operators may have different strengths and capabilities. Some may be strong punchers, while others excel with infighting, throwing, or takedowns. The krav maga system is designed to best conform to defenders. A defender does not have to compromise his capabilities to conform to any set solutions or prescribed movements. To adopt and streamline the krav maga method, you must personalize the techniques and make them your own. This begins conceptually and ends tactically. Choose the ballistic strikes and other combatives you feel most comfortable with and that give you the greatest confidence.

Krav Maga's Core Tenets

Make attacking the assailant instinctive. Target the assailant's anatomical vulnerabilities.

Train defense as simultaneous offense. Combine your defense and offense into one complete strategy.

Practice continuous combat motion. Krav maga emphasizes retzev, a Hebrew word that means "continuous motion." Combine and synchronize counterattack combatives in a logical way to overwhelm the assailant, giving your opponent little or no time to either react or recover.

Understand the difference between retzev and a mere series of counterattacks. A series of counterattacks lacks continuity; your counterviolence will not flow instinctively. Retzev enables your body to move instinctively—without thinking about your next move—in combat motion to exploit your assailant's vulnerabilities.

Take decisive action. Take him out.

Eliminate fighting inhibitions. Do whatever is necessary to overcome a dangerous threat. Damage—as opposed to hurt—your assailant.

Master a few effective tactics. Learn a few core defensive movements and counterattacks.

Make your training as real as possible. Training must attempt to simulate a real attack for you to understand the speed, ferocity, and strength a determined assailant may direct at you.

Visualize and plan scenarios. In addition to training with a partner, you can also use your mind to train your body to automatically and instinctively react to danger.

Krav Maga Tactical Positioning

Footwork and body positioning, whether standing or prone, allow you to simultaneously defend and attack, leading to seamless combative transitions essential to retzev. The key to evasion is moving out of the "line of fire" or the path of an opponent's offensive combatives. Clearly, positioning yourself where you can counterattack your opponent more easily than he can attack you is most advantageous. It is self-evident that fight positioning determines your tactical advantage. Optimally, a skilled krav maga fighter will move quickly to a superior and dominant position relative to his opponent, known in krav maga parlance as the deadside.

The deadside often provides you with a decisive tactical advantage. This strategy should revolve around your capabilities and preferred tactics involving long, medium, and short combatives combined with evasive maneuvers. Positioning becomes even more important when facing multiple assailants. Once superior position is achieved, the opponent will have minimal ability to defend or to counter your retzev attack. Remember, retzev, because it uses all parts of your body and incorporates multiple facets of fighting, provides an overwhelming counterattack.

When facing multiple assailants, you must only engage one at a time, using optimum combatives and movement while putting that opponent between you and any others. Inexperienced assailants will fortunately group together. If the student uses correct tactical positioning (never between two assailants), he limits the assailants' abilities to harm him. There is a limitation on how many assailants can occupy the same space to get at you. In select circumstances, you may have to go through them. (Krav maga has techniques for this.)

Reacting to an Ambush

Reacting from surprise allows the use of more force because you do not have time to rationally or reasonably analyze the situation. In other words, you are reacting defensively and catching up necessarily within fractions of a second to calibrate your response. Again, krav maga's goal is to have you react instantaneously without thinking. To reiterate, the overriding essence of krav maga is to neutralize an assailant immediately. The moment you are deemed safe, any additional defensive actions may, in fact, become offensive actions. If you continue to injure an assailant who is no longer a threat, you could face civil and criminal charges—especially if you deliberately turn the assailant's weapon on him.

Five Elements of an Ambush

1. Ambush victims are usually distracted, complacent, outnumbered, or caught in a state of maximum unpreparedness (negative five).

2. Victims' chances of escape are minimized or nonexistent since the assailant has chosen the site and circumstances.

3. Assailants often act from some sort of concealment or close in on their unwitting victims.

4. Assailants give themselves a way to escape.

5. Assailants have the intent—and usually the capability—to dominate their victims.

Seeing an Attack

Blind spots inhibit human vision. Therefore, a low-line kick or uppercut-type strike may come in under the visual radar. Human vision is also limited in judging the speed from an attack coming straight on and recognizing the speed of something traveling against a static background. Therefore, tactically, straight attacks are more difficult to recognize and defend. Oblong attacks such as hooks and roundhouse kicks are, accordingly, more recognizable. In addition, these looping types of attacks, by their nature, have to travel roughly three times the distance of a linear attack.

Trained fighters look for the mental commitment and corresponding physical manifestations such as blood draining from the face, increased breathing, and a subtle weight shift forward before the actual physical attack. While pupil dilation and constriction can indicate an impending attack, an experienced fighter may attack you without these phenomena, precisely because he has done it before and it has become second nature. One strong indicator is a head-to-toe slight shudder as adrenaline pours into his system. If he contracts his frame rather than expanding it, you may be dealing with a trained fighter coiling to spring into action.

Importantly, it is widely accepted that roughly eighty-five percent or more of the world's population is right handed and, therefore, right-side dominant. The majority of attacks are likely to be initiated by an attacker using his right arm. Nevertheless, it is crucial to train against all contingencies, including attacks initiated with the left hand. A skilled fighter will use all of his limbs in various combinations and may change his stance repeatedly to gain an advantage. Yet, the majority of unskilled or semiskilled attackers will initiate from their strong side. When training, we suggest taking this consideration into account. This can become especially important when closing on someone to put him into dominant control by controlling his favored arm.

The Language of Krav Maga

Throughout *Krav Maga Professional Tactics*, the following terms will appear frequently. Once you understand the language of krav maga, you can better understand the method.

Cavalier: A wrist takedown forcing an adversary's wrist to move against its natural range of motion, usually combined with tai-sabaki for added power.

Cold weapons: Blunt and edged weapons.

Combative: Any manner of strike, takedown, throw, joint lock, choke, or other offensive fighting movement.

Deadside: Your adversary's deadside, in contrast to his liveside, places you behind his near shoulder or facing his back. You are in an advantageous position to counterattack and control him because it is difficult for him to use his arm and leg farthest away from you to attack you. You should always move to the deadside when possible. When executed properly, this will also place the adversary between you and any third-party threat.

Elbow kiss: When securing an edged weapon or firearm held by an assailant and pinning it against his body, the defender moves to the assailant's deadside, creating an angle between the defender's arm and assailant's arm where the tips of their elbows touch or "kiss." The defender's forearm and assailant's gun arm create a "V" by the underside of the defender's forearm pressing against the topside of the assailant's forearm.

Figure four: A control hold securing an adversary's arm, torso, or ankle to exert pressure. The hold is performed by using both of your arms on the joint of the wrist, shoulder, or tendon of an adversary. For example, say you have secured your adversary's right wrist (his elbow is pointed toward the ground) with your right hand placed on the flat of his right hand, bending his wrist inward, with his elbow (tip toward the ground) pinned to your chest. At the same time, you simultaneously slip your other arm over the top of his forearm to interlock his arm and grab your own forearm. This positional arm control may also be used to attack the Achilles tendon with the blade of your forearm or control an adversary's torso from the rear mount. A figure four may also be applied to an adversary's torso by hooking one leg across the torso and securing it in the crook of the other knee.

Glicha: A sliding movement on the balls of your feet to carry your entire body weight forward and through a combative strike to maximize its impact.

Green zone: Major muscle groups of the limbs. Green-zone strikes are designed to distract and provide a temporary debilitating effect.

Gunt: Angled elbow block defense.

Hot weapons: Firearms.

Inside defense: An inside defense defends against an inside or straight attack. This type of attack involves a thrusting motion such as jabbing your finger into someone's eye or punching someone in the nose.

Kravist: A term I coined to describe a smart and prepared krav maga fighter.

Left outlet stance: Blade your body by turning your feet approximately 30 degrees to your right, with your left arm and left leg forward. (You can also turn 30 degrees to your right to come into a right regular outlet stance so that your right leg and arm are forward.) One may modify the stance for comfort's sake, perhaps by angling the rear foot at more than 30 degrees or in whatever way allows for quickest movement. Rest on both balls of your feet in a comfortable and balanced position. Your feet should be parallel, with about 55 percent of your weight distributed over your front leg. Your arms are positioned in front of your face and bent slightly forward at approximately a 60-degree angle between your forearms and your upper arms. From this stance, you will move forward, laterally, and backward, moving your feet in concert.

Liveside: When you are in front of your adversary and your adversary can both see you and use all four arms and legs against you, you are facing his or her liveside.

Nearside: Your adversary's limb closest to your torso.

Negative five: You are caught unaware and at a complete disadvantage. The assailant has the advantage of surprise and positioning.

Off angle: An attack angle that is not face to face.

Inoperable weapon: This occurs when a live round is partially lodged and improperly secured in the firing chamber of a firearm that loads automatically.

Outside defense: An outside defense counters an outside attack, that is, an attack directed at you from the outside of your body to the inside. A slap to the face or hook punch are examples of outside attacks.

Personal weapons: Hands, feet, elbows, knees, body limbs, head, and teeth.

Retzev: A Hebrew word that means "continuous motion" in combat. Retzev, the backbone of modern Israeli krav maga, teaches you to move your body instinctively in combat motion without thinking about your next move. When in a dangerous situation, you'll automatically call upon your physical and mental training to launch a seamless, overwhelming counterattack using strikes, takedowns, throws, joint locks, chokes, or other offensive actions combined with evasive action. Retzev is quick and decisive movement, merging all aspects of your krav maga training. Defensive movements transition automatically into offensive movements to neutralize the attack, affording your adversary little time to react.

Same side: Your same-side arm or leg faces your adversary when you are positioned opposite one another. For example, if you are directly facing your adversary and your right side is opposite your adversary's left side, your same-side arm is your right arm (opposite his left arm).

Secoul: A larger step than glicha, covering more distance to carry your entire body weight forward and through a combative strike to maximize its impact.

Stepping off the line: Using footwork and body movement to take evasive action against a linear attack such as a straight punch or kick. Such movement is also referred to as **breaking the angle of attack**.

Red zone: The head, spine, vital organs, and groin. Red-zone strikes are designed to shock the attacker's central nervous system and stop his movements.

Tai-sabaki: A 180-degree or semicircle step by rotating one leg back to create torque on a joint to complete a takedown or control hold.

Trapping: Occurs when you pin or grab the adversary's arms with one arm leaving you free to continue combatives with your other arm.

CHAPTER 2

Defending the Most Common Upper-Body and Lower-Body Attacks, Throws, and Counterthrows

Footwork and body positioning combined with timing, whether standing or prone, allow you to simultaneously defend and attack, leading to seamless combative transitions essential to retzev. The key to evasion is moving out of the "line of fire," or the path of an opponent's attack. In defending an assault or threat, krav maga's essential philosophy is for the defender to close the distance and neutralize the threat. Clearly, positioning yourself where you can counterattack your opponent more easily than he can attack you is most advantageous.

Optimally, the distance between the defender and the assailant can be closed before the assailant can

1. orchestrate the assault to debilitate the adversary with strong combatives,

2. deny the assailant access to any weapon, and

3. achieve dominant control.

If a weapon is successfully deployed and put into action, closing the distance allows the defender to either deflect-redirect or parry the weapon in conjunction with body defenses while delivering withering counterattacks.

Most advantageously, a kravist will automatically move quickly to a superior and dominant position relative to his adversary, known in krav maga parlance as the deadside. Achieving deadside positioning often provides a decisive tactical advantage, especially when the defender can deploy a cold or hot weapon in addition to his personal weapons. Your finishing strategy should revolve around your capabilities and preferred tactics involving long, medium, and short combatives combined with evasive maneuvers and weapon deployment. Positioning becomes even more important when facing multiple adversaries.

Straight-Punch Defenses

As emphasized, krav maga combines, whenever possible, a deflection with a body defense to avoid an attack (including those with a weapon) and uses retzev counterattacks to neutralize the threat. Your defensive hand used to deflect the strike should always lead your body. In other words, your arm deflection should precede the rest of your body's defensive movement by fractions of a second. This gets you out of the line of fire or "off the line" to provide a double layer of protection, redirecting a threat while at the same moment moving yourself away from the threat. The following are select defenses and combinations.

Note: there are terminal applications of force not represented here. We train military units in these techniques and will only do so in person. Please contact us at david@israeli krav.com for more information.

Sliding Parry with Eye Strike

This defense allows you to deflect an incoming rear punch or cross while delivering a nearly simultaneous same-side eye strike.

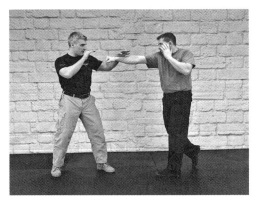

Parry the strike with your palm heel or lower forearm. *Attack* the assailant's incoming arm with your deflection.

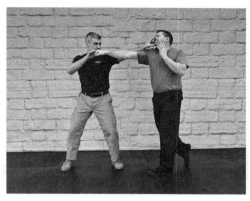

Use your same-side arm to immediately strike the assailant's eyes. It is an "opener" for you to continue retzev combatives.

Sliding Parry While Stepping Off the Line

This defense allows you to deflect an incoming rear punch or cross while simultaneously moving slightly away from the punch as you deliver your own counterattack strike to the throat, chin, nose, midsection, or groin. Note that this defense and the following related defenses enable a defender to use the same defense (albeit with opposite movements) against a straight punch to close on the assailant and neutralize the threat. Your hand leads your body defense to redirect the adversary's punch by sliding down your adversary's right arm while your right arm delivers a half-roundhouse counterpunch to the throat, chin, or nose.

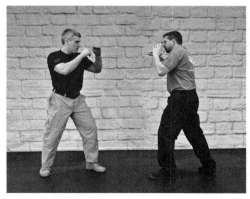

Defending from your left outlet stance.

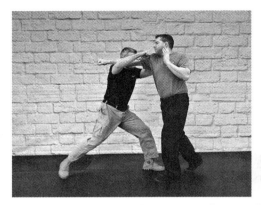 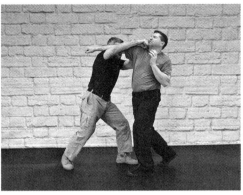

Step to your left while bringing your left cupped hand diagonally across your face close to your right shoulder. The key is to deflect and step off the line, moving both feet together while simultaneously counterpunching. Do not lunge; keep your feet equidistant by moving them the same distance. You may also punch low to the assailant's body, targeting his liver, or deliver a hand strike to his groin. (These last two counterstrikes are useful if an assailant has a height advantage and you cannot readily reach his head to counterattack.)

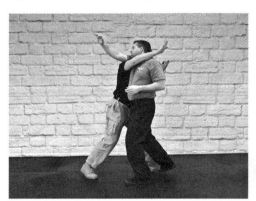 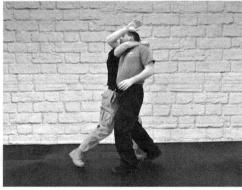

This defense is readily followed up with trapping the adversary's right arm and placing him in a standing triangle "blood choke." Be sure to secure his right shoulder tightly against his right carotid artery while using the radial bone of your right arm against his left carotid artery. You could also drop him to the ground with an *osoto-gari* type of takedown.

Modified Standing Triangle Choke

Slip your counterpunch arm around the assailant's neck, placing your biceps against one side of the main arteries. These arteries, the common right and left carotids, carry blood to the brain through the carotid sheath. Trapping the assailant's shoulder against the other side of the main arteries, clamp down in a figure four to execute a blood choke. Lastly, a number of strong takedowns are available from this triangular choke position, including taking the assailant down into formidable choke positions on the ground. In addition, there are number of devastating throws one may use to break the assailant from the modified triangle hold.

Notes:

1. For the sliding parry defense, if you misread the assailant's straight punch—for instance, he throws a left punch instead of a right—stepping off the line properly will still allow the defense to work. You will have avoided the punch with a body defense (stepping off the line of attack) while counterattacking. In essence, you will "split" the assailant's hands with your counterpunch. The immediate danger is that you are still to your adversary's liveside: he still may have the ability to mount an effective counterattack. *The preferred defense is always to move to his deadside, minimizing his ability to counterattack.*

2. The inside sliding-parry defenses can be used when the defender is on the ground and slightly on his side. The assailant is braced against your topside shin with your other heel on his leg or hip to keep him at bay (sometimes known as the modified "Z guard"). The key is a strong body defense moving away or deadside to the punch with a proper slide and simultaneous counterpunch into a choke hold. Be sure to slide fully up his attacking arm as you simultaneously counter-strike using an eye rake or punch. This will set up additional combatives, including (but not limited to) a short hook to the head or throat, and also position you on your side for a straight armbar.

3. These sliding defenses may also be used with great effect against outside sucker punches if the assailant is slightly in front of you. The finishes can be the same as described previously. Timing—as with all defenses—is crucial. You must step out of the line of attack in time to deflect and counterpunch.

Two-Handed Sliding Parry with Knee Counterattack

This is a devastating counterattack using a two-handed deflection and body defense combined with a knee counterattack to the assailant's groin or midsection.

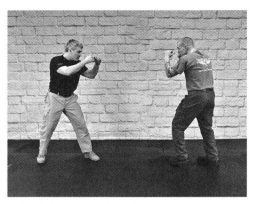

Defend from the left outlet stance.

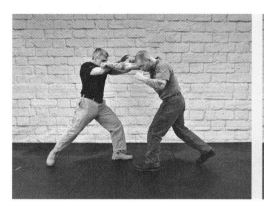 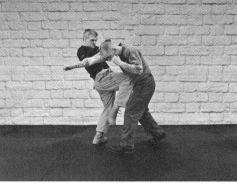

Use both arms to deflect the adversary's incoming straight right punch. Turn both of your arms so that the forearms are facing in the same direction with your hands slightly cupped, palms down. This allows for a strong sliding deflection against the outside of your adversary's right arm. You must again step off the line to your left. As you step, propel your knee with your body weight behind it into your adversary's groin or midsection with a modified roundhouse knee.

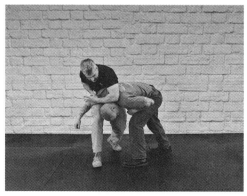

Follow up with an over-the-top elbow, slamming down on the back of your adversary's neck combined with additional retzev combatives.

Note: you may also use a variation of this defense if your assailant attempts to "sucker punch" you and you are both facing the same direction. Once again you must step off the line and with a double forearm parry to deliver a powerful roundhouse knee to his midsection.

Inside "L" Parry against a Straight Rear Punch While Stepping Off the Line into Irimi Strike and Hanging Choke

This defense, similar to the inside sliding parry, allows you to deflect an incoming straight right punch from either side while simultaneously moving away from the punch, trapping your adversary's arm, and delivering an *irimi* strike into a hanging choke hold position. The parrying movement covers no more than six inches and will lead the defensive body movement. It is important to note that this is not an uncontrolled swipe or grab at the assailant's incoming arm (a common mistake when first learning the technique). The length of the defensive arm from the pinky to the elbow is used to deflect any change in the height of the adversary's strike. The movement rotates the left wrist outward so your left thumb, which is kept alongside the palm with all the fingers pointing up, turns away from you as contact is made with the adversary's arm to redirect his incoming strike.

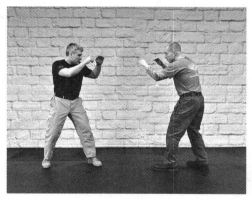

Defend from the left outlet stance.

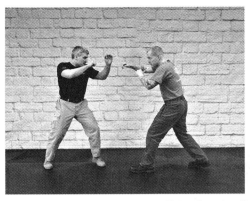 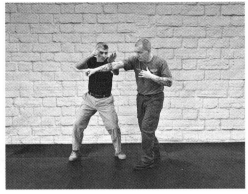

Using proper footwork, move off the line, leading the body defense with your left parry.

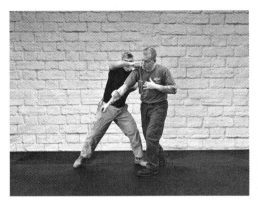 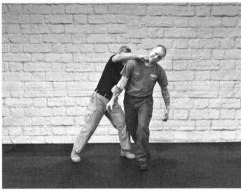

After parrying, hook the assailant's arm by cupping your left hand and pinning down the arm against the assailant's torso while delivering a counterpunch to the throat or jaw.

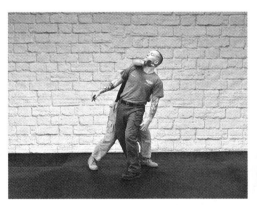 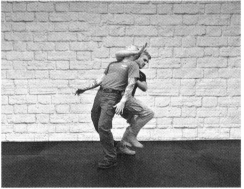

Once you have stunned the assailant, bend your elbow slightly and extend your forearm (using the radius) to deliver an irimi clothesline combative into a standing choke facilitated by "popping" the opponent's back forward with your left arm. Note: you may omit the initial strike and deliver the irimi strike right away. Keep your striking arm slightly bent to prevent your elbow from hyperextending. Strike the opponent's throat and then step through for the choke.

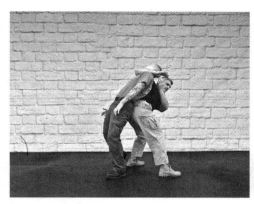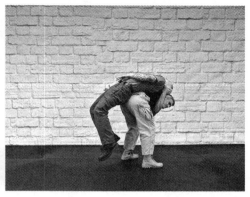

Maintaining tight control, step around the opponent and secure his neck in the crook of your arm. Cinch the choke and thrust your hips into the assailant, lifting him from the ground and loading your hips properly. *These hanging technique variations are only to be used in a life-and-death situation.*

Note: this defense is also used against a straight stab with an elongated weapon.

Hook-Punch Defenses

Hook-Punch Defense into Control #6

This technique demonstrates the instinctive nature of krav maga by harnessing one's natural response of flinching and "swatting" away an incoming attack. Importantly, however, you are not swatting away his incoming arm as much as attacking it with an outside chopping movement.

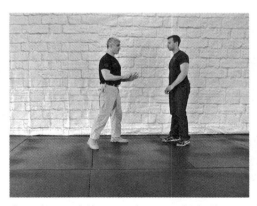

Defending from an interview, de-escalation, or when caught in the negative five.

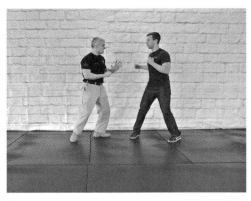 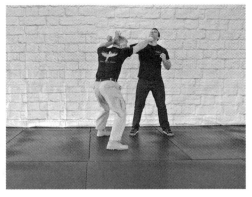

Block and attack his incoming punch with the underside (ulnar bone) of your nearside arm against the assailant's incoming strike as you simultaneously step off the line of attack while punching to the assailant's jaw or windpipe. This combative must be justified, as it has the potential to seriously injure an adversary.

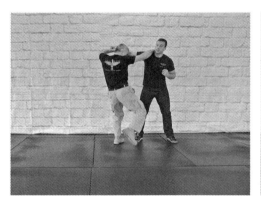 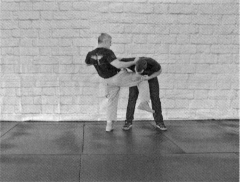

Secure his attacking arm at the wrist while delivering a straight knee to the thigh (green zone) or, if necessary, to the groin (red zone). See below.

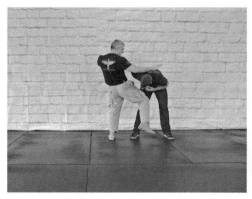 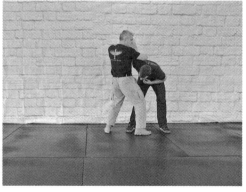

Seize control of the assailant's arm by the right wrist. With your free arm, slam the top of your forearm (radial bone) into the crook of the assailant's elbow to fold it, allowing a Control #6 (*kimura* lock).

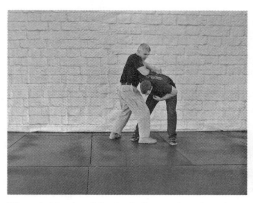 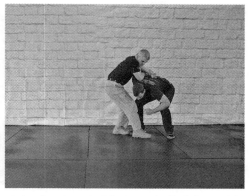

Wrench his shoulder both forward and up to assert dominant control for a controlled descent to the ground. Be sure to keep the assailant's shoulder and torso pressed to your body to assert dominant control.

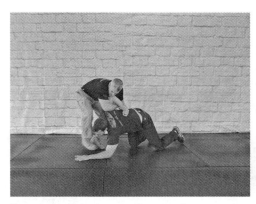 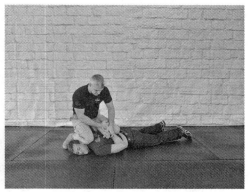

Forcefully slide the assailant to the ground to your two o'clock (to prevent him from rolling or resisting). If appropriate, apply restraints.

"Instinctive" Hook-Punch Double-Block Defense

This technique demonstrates once again the instinctive nature of krav maga by harnessing one's natural response of flinching or placing two arms up to shield the upper body.

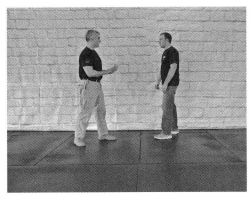 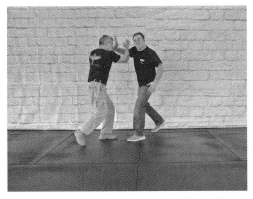

Defend from an interview or de-escalation position, or when caught in the negative five. Simultaneously intercept the punch with both arms bent about 60 degrees, making contact with the underside of your arms (ulnar bones) against the assailant's incoming strike.

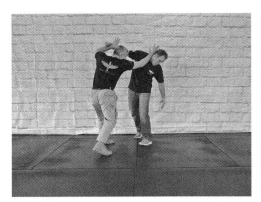 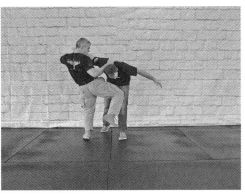

Immediately use a chop to the carotid sheath. Follow up with additional combatives, including a straight knee to the thigh (green zone) or, if necessary, (not depicted) to the groin (red zone).

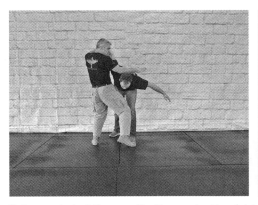 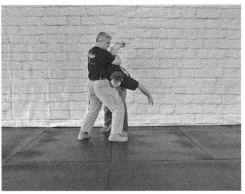

Seize control of the assailant's arm by the right wrist. With your free arm, slam the top of your forearm (radial bone) into the crook of the assailant's elbow to fold it, allowing a Control #6 (kimura lock).

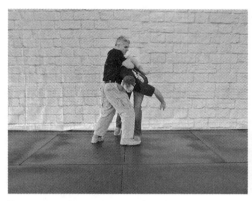 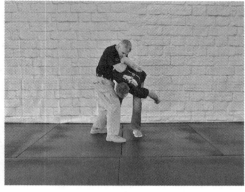

Be sure to keep the assailant's shoulder and torso pressed to your body to assert dominant control. You have the option of sliding the assailant to the ground at your two o'clock (to prevent him from rolling or resisting) and then applying restraints. See Hook-Punch Defense into Control #6.

Hook-Punch Defense with Face Control into Choke

This technique demonstrates the continuous combat flow of krav maga by defending one of the most common attacks, a hook punch.

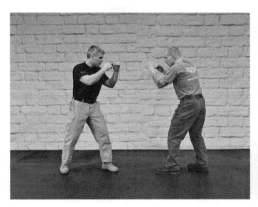 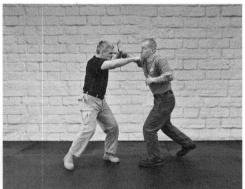

From your left outlet stance, move off the line of attack as you execute a 360 rotational outside block and counterpunch.

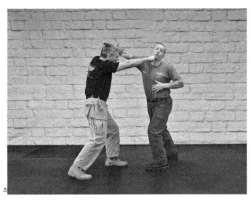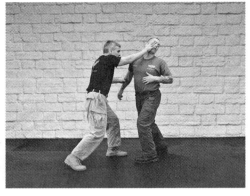

Simultaneously parry and attack using a straight punch, web strike to the throat (using the web of the hand to strike the Adam's apple), palm heel, or other option. Maintain contact with your parrying arm and force the arm down while using your free hand to cross-face him with your fingers in his nearside eye.

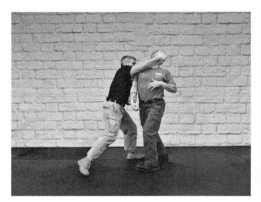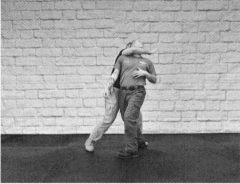

Continue to apply pressure to his face as you maneuver to take his back.

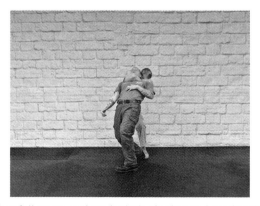

Execute the choke. Other follow-up options include ripping and tearing the assailant's face. You may also clinch the face from the rear to sprawl your adversary backward with the option of a knee to the base of the skull or spine.

Hook-Punch Defense with Spin into Face Control

This is another technique that demonstrates the continuous combat flow of krav maga.

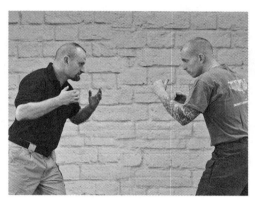

Defend from your left outlet stance.

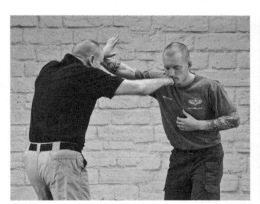
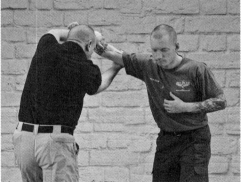

Move off the line of attack as you execute a 360 rotational outside instinctive block and counterpunch.

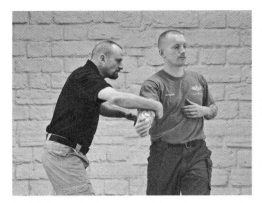 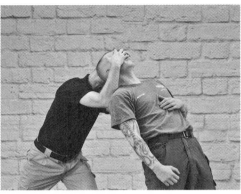

Maintain contact with your blocking arm and reach underneath the adversary's elbow to secure it with a cupped hook, just below the crook. Keep your thumb alongside your palm rather than clasp his arm with your thumb. Execute the face control.

Hook-Punch Defense with Spin into Choke

Similar to the previous technique, this technique places the defender in a position to execute a rear choke.

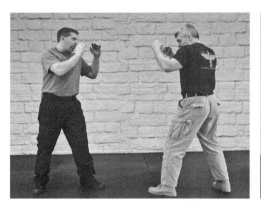 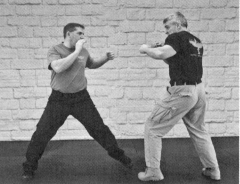

From your left outlet stance, move off the line of attack as you execute a 360 rotational outside block and counterpunch, web strike to the throat, palm heel, or other option.

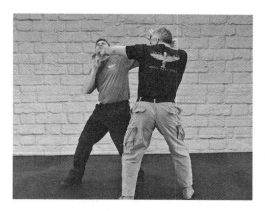

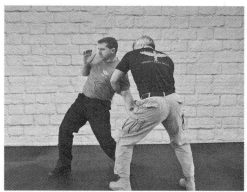

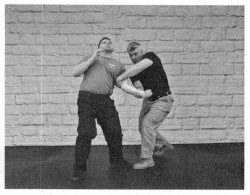

Maintain contact with your blocking arm and reach underneath the adversary's elbow to secure it with a cupped hook, just below the crook. Keep your thumb alongside your palm rather than clasp his arm with your thumb. Reach underneath his elbow and pull your adversary back to you with both hands, using tai-sabaki footwork to spin his torso and position him with his back to you.

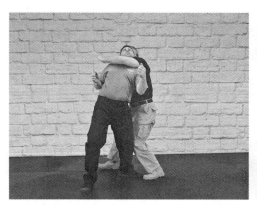

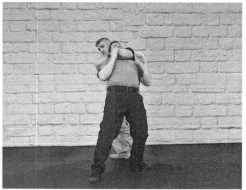

Execute the choke. Other follow-up options include ripping and tearing the assailant's face by inserting fingers ("fishhooks") into your adversary's eyes and clawing the face and throat. You may also clinch the face from the rear to sprawl your adversary backward with the option of a knee to the base of the skull or spine.

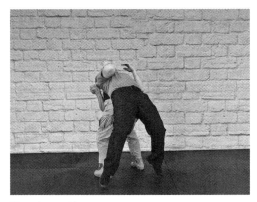

Hanging option.

Choke Holds

Chokes are fight enders. Chokes must only be used in a self-defense situation where you have an acute fear that the assailant intends you serious bodily harm. In krav maga parlance, there are two types of choke holds, "chokes" and "blood chokes." Both techniques achieve the same result: unconsciousness, brain damage, or death, depending on the force and length of time for which the choke is applied.

Chokes cut off the oxygen supply to the brain by preventing air from refilling the lungs. In addition, a choke can cause severe damage to the trachea, hyoid bone, and larynx. (Be aware that a choke or strangulation technique can exacerbate or trigger a preexisting medical condition, resulting in death.) The tongue can also become lodged in the back of the throat and occlude airflow.

Blood chokes or strangulation techniques stop the flow of blood by constricting the carotid artery and jugular veins on the sides of the neck that carry oxygenated and deoxygenated blood. As emphasized, you must not allow anyone to get his or her hands, arms, or legs around your neck.

Choke techniques can utilize the hands, forearms, or other objects such as a stick or rolled-up magazine placed across the throat. The key to proper chokes is using your hands and arms to provide leverage and compression that leave your adversary few, if any, defenses. The narrower the choking implement, the easier the insertion under the adversary's chin to attack the neck.

The ulnar and radial edges of the wrist and forearm are particularly well suited to apply compression to the throat and neck. An adversary's clothing can be used against him, and so can yours—so beware. You must keep your head close to your adversary to avoid countertechniques. The following three techniques are applied from the rear, the most advantageous choking position.

This **"professional" rear naked choke** can be thought of as a superior combination of the two previous choking techniques because of the extreme pressure that may be applied. The blade of the forearm and biceps apply pressure to the adversary's carotid sheath on both sides of the neck, stopping blood flow to his brain. Grab your left biceps with your right hand. Snake the nonchoking arm behind your adversary's head and place your hand on the rear of his skull. Do not place the hand too high because the adversary can remove or pluck it away to disable the choke. To apply pressure, squeeze your choking arm toward you and flex your nonchoking arm's biceps while exerting pressure forward with your hand clenched in a fist. At the same time, lean the side of your head into your hand for added choking pressure.

Your body is essentially both leaning forward (on the top plane of your left arm) and pulling back (on the bottom plane of your right arm) to exert maximum choking pressure. To optimize the choke, you may rock the assailant slightly to one side and then the other to cinch the choke and thwart his counters. Keep your body tight to your adversary and tuck your head. Clasp your hand with your nonchoking arm and squeeze your arms together to constrict blood flow. This choke is highly effective. You should keep your hips square for the opportunity to apply the choke with either arm. When on the ground, do not cross your hooked feet unless you can obtain a figure-four position and keep your legs on your adversary's thighs to prevent him from applying ankle locks.

The **crook-of-the-elbow hanging choke**—a blood choke—applies pressure to the adversary's carotid sheath on both sides of the neck. This pressure occludes blood flow to his brain. Pressure is applied using your biceps muscle and radius of the arm. Keep your body tight to your adversary with your head tucked. Clasp your right hand with your left hand and squeeze your arms together to constrict blood flow. When practicing with a partner, use extreme caution.

Flooring an Assailant

You can put an assailant on the ground in three ways:

1. *Undermine his balance.* Combatives include strikes, throwing.

2. *Undermine his support.* Combatives include strikes, trips, and leg sweeps, especially on the front leg as he moves forward and shifts his weight.

3. *Lock his joints to force him down.* When the defender is still standing, a heel hook is especially effective. The heel hook is best applied by using your hip and core, not just your leg. As you move your hip, drag your leg with you to ensnare the leg while knocking his torso off balance.

Keep in mind that a defender often falls to the ground with an assailant as the assailant grabs or locks on to him while falling. Flailing and grabbing are natural instincts when falling to the ground. Do these both strategically and tactically to attack his vulnerabilities—eyes, throat, groin.

To control an adversary's center of gravity, a push or pull move is usually used. This type of combative is best used when perpendicular to the adversary's center of gravity (as in, not at an angle when either of his legs can easily recover to restore his balance). The goal is to remove both his support and balance simultaneously.

The Israeli krav maga curriculum incorporates a number of throws. Founder Imi Lichtenfeld was awarded a black belt in judo by Moshe Feldenkrais, who trained in Japan directly under the legendary Kano Jigoro. Selecting a throw is obviously determined by body positioning and the dynamics of the entry for the throw. The goal with throws and takedowns, as with all krav maga thinking, is to accomplish the greatest effect with the least effort.

The formula is simple: krav maga is designed to overcome any disparities in size or strength. The key, once again, is simultaneous attack and defense to disrupt the attack and immediately redirect it into a throw or takedown, using gravity and the ground to further neutralize the threat. A strong combative will stun the assailant, allowing you to enter and unbalance him so you can complete the takedown or throw.

An unbalanced adversary is obviously easier to displace than a balanced one. Even if your initial throw or takedown is unsuccessful and the assailant maintains partial balance, you must continue with the retzev concept of continuous combat motion, applying a subsequent combative or series of combatives to keep attacking the threat. Always attempt to keep your retzev seamless, transitioning from one technique to another in a logical manner.

At the green-belt level (third belt level in the traditional krav maga curriculum), Imi incorporated several of judo's most accessible and effective throws and takedowns. In choosing these throws and takedowns, Imi married these techniques with many of the core defenses against upper-body attacks. In letting gravity take its course, coupled with momentum generated by the throw or takedown, Imi recognized that slamming someone into the ground would help take the fight out of him—or, at the least, momentarily diminish his offensive capabilities.

When an assailant attempts to throw you, by the very nature of movement and tactics, he is creating an opening for you to counterthrow. (This is true of all combatives, including kicking, punching, knees, and elbows. A good fighter will minimize these openings, but they are still there to be exploited if the defender is skilled enough to recognize and execute the countertechnique properly.)

The following throws and takedowns are designed for professionals wearing law enforcement and military combat gear. These tactics are specifically designed to help keep, as much as possible, the professional kravist from becoming entangled with the assailant. In addition, these techniques account for the extra weight load or displacement and mobility restriction this type of gear places on the kravist. *Each of the following throws assumes the defender is on the assailant's right side and has just defended a right straight punch.* Included are the Japanese names for these takedowns and throws, as these are transliterated the same in the Israeli krav maga curriculum.

No-Rules Countertactics

In developing krav maga for the Israeli military, founder Imi Lichtenfeld recognized the need to account for and counter other military hand-to-hand combat systems, especially those relying heavily on judo. Accordingly, Imi developed krav maga–oriented ("no rules") countertactics. A few key techniques are included in the green-belt through advanced black-belt levels of the Israeli krav maga curriculum.

For counterthrows, you can take advantage of the assailant's momentum and displacement. In other words, by attempting to throw you, your assailant creates an opening for you to counterthrow. Importantly, this is true of all combatives, including kicking, punching, knees, elbows—all types of strikes. A good fighter will minimize these openings, but they are still there to be exploited if the defender is skilled enough to recognize them and execute the countertactic properly. Keep in mind that counterthrows are not without risk, since you have let the adversary somehow seize the initiative. Obviously, to be a good counterthrower, you must understand the principles and tactics of each throw.

Defending a Hook Punch into Throws

The following throws may be used after initially defending a hook punch. The same throwing principles apply as covered in the previous straight-punch sliding defenses using the transliterated Japanese names:

- Koshi guruma
- Harai goshi
- Ippon seoi nage

Hook-Punch Defense into Koshi Guruma

The 360 defense combined with stepping off the line of attack to the outside facilitates the *koshi guruma* throw. After initially blocking the punch while stepping offline to stun the assailant, you can apply koshi guruma (hip wheel throw) by using the correct footwork and turning your torso into the assailant. Do not begin the throwing action until you have the assailant off balance by forcing his weight decidedly forward over his feet.

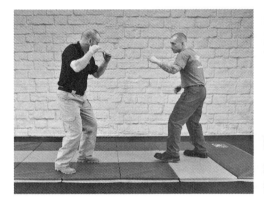 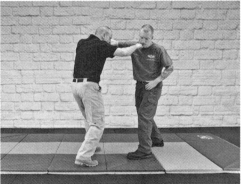

Defend from your left outlet stance. Step off the line while blocking and counterattacking.

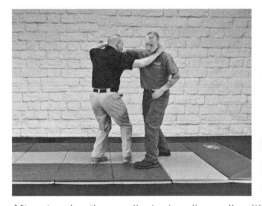 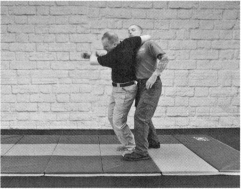

After stunning the assailant, step diagonally with your right foot to the inside of the assailant's (right) foot. As you crossover step, begin angling your body and slide the left heel to the inside of the assailant's (left) nearside foot. These two entry steps turn your back into the assailant's torso. Your (right) hip must be positioned outside of the assailant's (right) hip. Pull the assailant's right arm straight out and around you to unbalance him to his right front while your right arm simultaneously pulls him forward toward you, creating a whipsaw effect. Your bodies must be glued together with no slack.

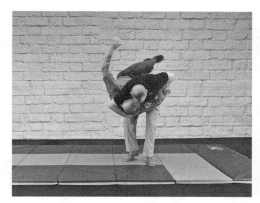 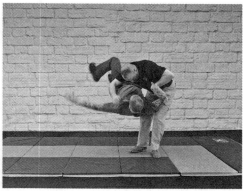

As you shift onto the ball of your left foot, simultaneously pull forward quickly with your left arm, moving in a circular motion. To throw the assailant, bend your knees to obtain leverage, with your hips below the assailant's hips. As you pull the assailant forward, shift your weight onto the balls of your feet, slightly flexing your knees for balance. Be sure to tightly control his upper body. Squeeze tightly, straighten your legs, and rotate your torso by pulling forward in a decisive circular motion to rotate him over your right hip. This will allow you to upend him and smash him into the ground.

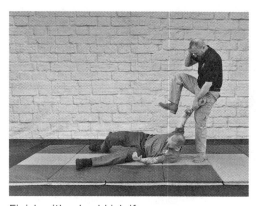

Finish with a heel kick if necessary.

Hook-Punch Defense into Harai Goshi

Similar to the previous two throws, after initially parrying the punch while stepping offline to stun the assailant, you can apply *harai goshi* (sweeping hip throw) by using the correct footwork and turning your torso into the assailant. Do not begin the sweeping action until the assailant is off balance, his weight forced decidedly forward over his right foot. Note again, for this throw, rock the assailant to your right corner to initially unbalance him. Keep the assailant tight to your torso. This assists the pull as you execute the throw.

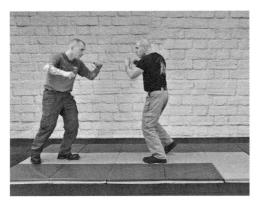 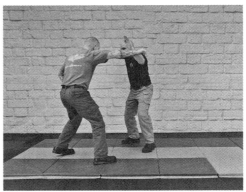

Defend from your left outlet stance. Step off the line while blocking and counterattacking.

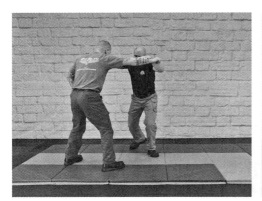 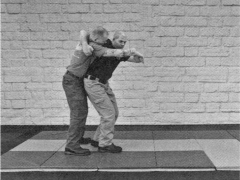

After stunning the assailant, step diagonally with your right foot to the inside of the assailant's (right) foot. As you step, begin angling your body and slide your left heel to the inside of the assailant's (left) nearside foot. These two entry steps turn your back into the assailant's torso. Your (right) hip must be positioned slightly outside of the assailant's (right) hip. Pull the assailant's right arm straight out and around you to unbalance him to his right front corner while your right arm simultaneously pulls him forward toward you, creating a whipsaw effect.

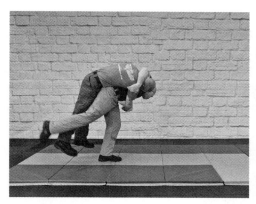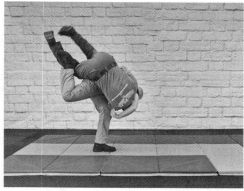

As you pull the assailant forward, shift your weight onto the ball of your left foot, slightly flexing your knee for balance. As you shift onto the ball of your left foot, simultaneously sweep your right leg back, scything the assailant's right lower leg. It is essential that you pull straight out into a circle with your left arm. As you pull forward and into the circular motion, line up your right leg to kick decisively backward with your toes down, using the inside of your calf muscle to scythe the outside of his lower leg, thereby sweeping the leg and smashing him to the ground.

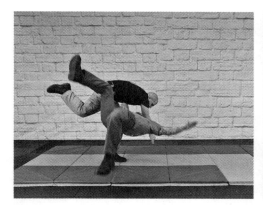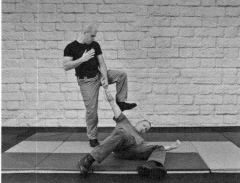

Sweep your right leg back with the toes pointed down while simultaneously driving your head and arms down to complete the throw. Deliver a heel kick if necessary.

Straight-Punch Defense into Ippon Seoi Nage ("Outside" One-Armed Shoulder Throw, Arm-Break Variation)

Ippon seoi nage is a throw tailor-made for this particular krav maga defense. After initially parrying the punch with an over-the-top sliding defense, you must quickly secure the assailant's punching arm. Naturally, he will retract the arm. Therefore, your over-the-top punch must stun him, allowing you to isolate his arm. While stepping off the line, simultaneously counterpunch and secure his arm with your free (rear) arm. Using the correct footwork while turning your torso into the assailant with proper body positioning, apply the Ippon Seoi Nage, Arm-Break Variation.

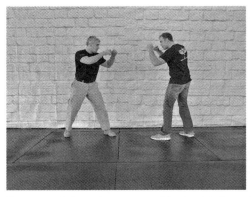 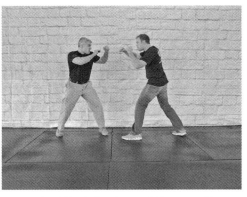

From your left outlet stance, sidestep his incoming punch while delivering a sliding over-the-top counterpunch. Keep your thumb pointed up, allowing your inverted punch to drive his arm down while sliding your arm atop of his to deliver the punch. You must stun the attacker because otherwise he will naturally retract his arm, thereby thwarting the throw attempt.

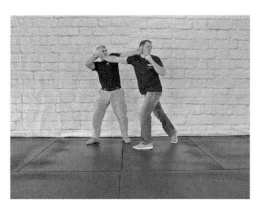 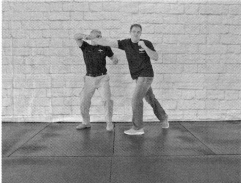

After you deliver the stunning blow to the assailant's head, secure the assailant's right arm and step forward with your left leg to turn your body 90 degrees to initiate the throw.

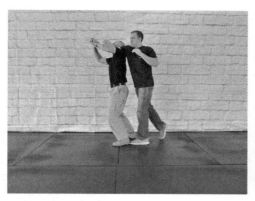 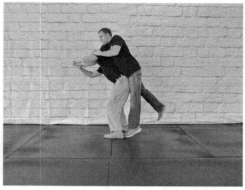

As you crossover step with your right foot to switch your stance and finish angling your body, simultaneously snake your left counterattack arm underneath the assailant's right arm *above his elbow joint*, fitting the V of your bent elbow snugly into his armpit. The trapezius and deltoid of your right side should be directly inside his arm with your left side extremely close to the assailant's front.

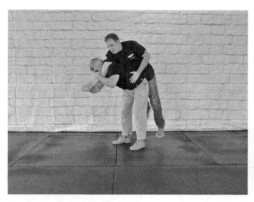 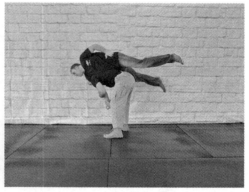

Keep the assailant's right arm secured with your left hand at his wrist. Bend your knees, positioning yourself with your hips in line with his groin or as low as possible and keeping your upper body straight to lift the assailant onto your back. If you wish to break the assailant's arm, secure his arm with his palm facing up to create an armbar that turns into an arm break. As you launch him, yank both of your hands down and to your right to jettison the assailant over your right shoulder.

Note: a variation of ippon seoi nage is to drop to one or both knees to hurl the assailant over your shoulder. Since you are closer to the ground (having dropped to your knees), the impact on the assailant may be less; nevertheless, this is an effective throw. The knee-drop variation may be used when a defender initially struggles or is forced forward.

Sliding Parry into Te Guruma (Hand Wheel or "Bucket Dump")

This defense allows you to deflect an incoming rear punch or cross while simultaneously moving away from the punch and delivering your own straight-punch counterattack to the throat, chin, nose, midsection, or groin. Note: this defense and the following related technique enable a defender to use the same defense (albeit with opposite movements) to counter a straight punch and close on the assailant to neutralize the threat.

The key is to deflect and step off the line, moving both feet together. Do not lunge; keep your feet equidistant by moving them the same distance. You may also punch low to the assailant's body, targeting his liver, or deliver a hand strike to his groin. (These last two counterstrikes are useful against assailants whose height advantage does not allow you to easily reach their head to counterattack.)

This defense is readily followed up by trapping the adversary's right arm and delivering a right straight knee to the groin or midsection, followed by a left over-the-top elbow (similar in movement to the over-the-top punch but instead using the elbow) to the back of the neck. Additional retzev combatives should follow, including multiple takedown options to land an adversary hard on his head. Once you dump him face first, continue with any additional combatives, such as heel stomps or taking his back, while administering punches or elbows to the back of his head or neck.

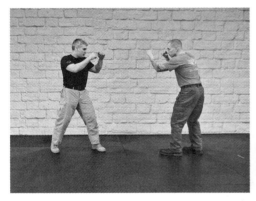 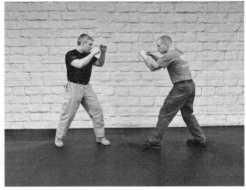

From your left outlet stance, step to your left while bringing your left cupped hand diagonally across your face, close to your right shoulder. Your hand will lead your body defense to redirect the adversary's punch by sliding down your adversary's right arm while your right arm delivers a half-roundhouse counterpunch to the throat, chin, or nose.

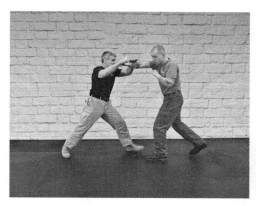 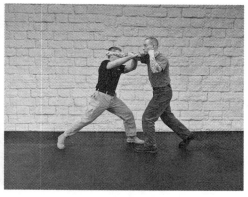

After you close the distance on your assailant with your simultaneous counterpunch, to execute te guruma, transition your punching arm to control his torso.

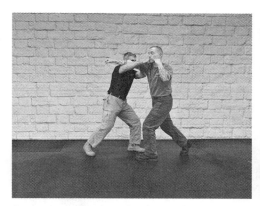 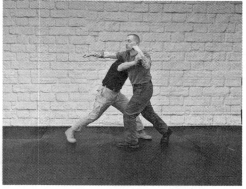

As you transition into the throw, sink your hips and thrust your other arm through the assailant's legs to first strike and then grab his groin.

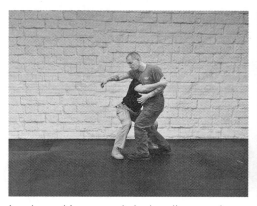 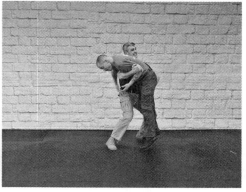

Load your hips properly by bending your knees with your back straight.

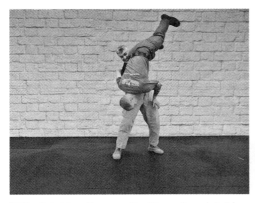
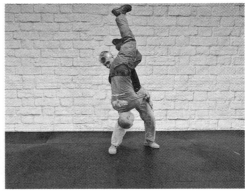

Still clutching the assailant's groin, pick him up to—in krav maga parlance—"bucket dump" him facedown or on his head.

Te Guruma Variation (Lurching the Assailant Forward)

The entry is the same as described above in Sliding Parry into Te Guruma (Hand Wheel or "Bucket Dump"). A variation of the throw is to forcefully lurch the assailant forward rather than pick him up. This variation demonstrates how krav maga is designed for smaller defenders, perhaps without the strength to pick up an attacker, to take him down nevertheless.

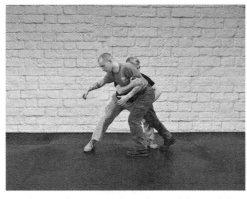
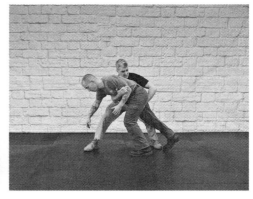

Load your hips properly and grab his testicles.

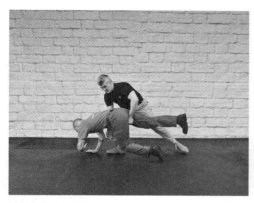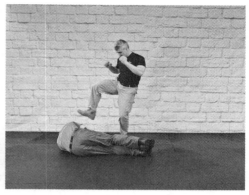

Make the "bucket scoop" motion without lifting the assailant high off the ground. Follow with kicks or other retzev combatives.

Counterthrows

As you evaluate the counterthrow techniques, keep in mind that counterthrows are not without risk, as you have let the adversary somehow seize the initiative. Obviously, to be a good counterthrower, you must understand the principles and tactics of each throw. Hence, Imi and Grandmaster Gidon's emphasis on learning core throwing techniques both for defensive and offensive purposes.

Hip Slide against a Throw

The key is to instantaneously ascertain a throw attempt and break hip contact with the assailant.

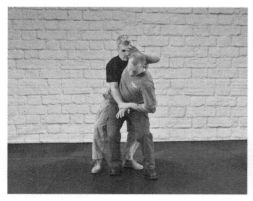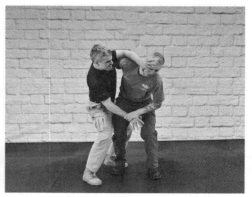

On recognizing or feeling an impending hand or leg throw, slide your hips off to the assailant's throw side.

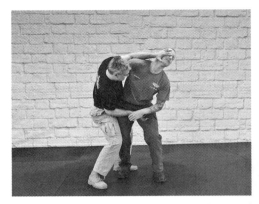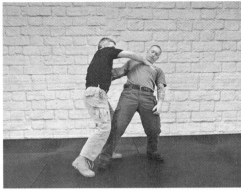

Attack the head with eye gouges or other combatives, including striking the throat.

Tani Otoshi (Valley Drop) against a Hand or Leg Throw

The *tani otoshi* defense is used to drop immediately when recognizing an impending hip or shoulder throw. The key, again, is to instantaneously ascertain a throw attempt and break hip contact by moving to the assailant's side while sinking your weight and strongly securing the assailant's waist.

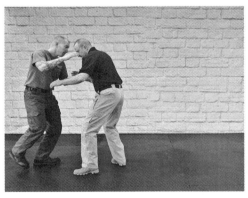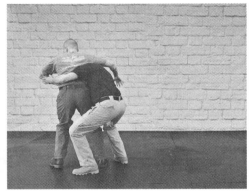

Immediately move to the side and sink your hips below the assailant's hips while splaying the opposite leg (the assailant's throw side) to prepare to whirl and smash the assailant into the ground.

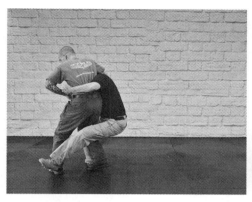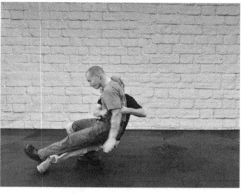

Once you quickly drop into position, pivot sharply to your splayed leg side (turning into the assailant) to smash the assailant's shoulder or head into the ground, driving your weight through the assailant.

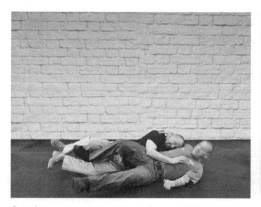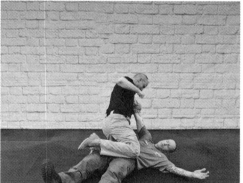

Continue your momentum into a high mount.

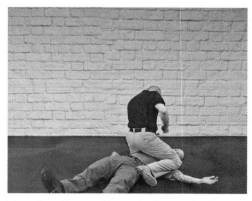

Pin the opponent's arm(s) and continue with combatives.

Straight-Punch Defense Using a Straight Kick

Use the longer range of the kick and timing to kick the assailant in the groin as he launches the punch.

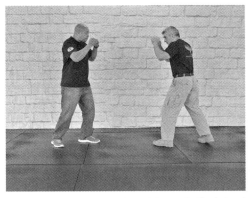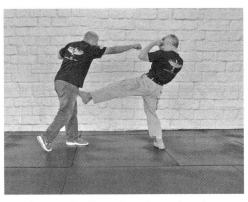

Use your front leg to kick with the ball of the foot to the assailant's groin or knee, keeping your hands up. Note: with more distance, you may also use a rear straight kick.

Core Kick Defenses

Shin Deflection against a Straight Kick

The shin deflection provides a proximate and natural defense against an assailant launching a low kick from either his front or rear leg.

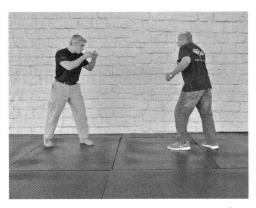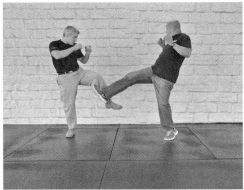

From your regular outlet stance, use your front leg or foot to deflect or parry an incoming kick without dropping your hands. Slide your front leg across your body while maintaining your balance, but do not overcommit your front leg, which may throw you off balance, and, more importantly, put you in a vulnerable position.

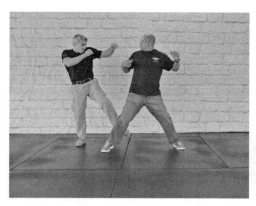 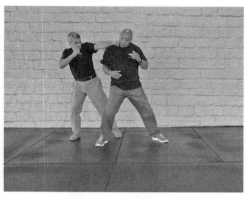

Once you have successfully parried the kick, continue your momentum forward into a straight lead punch counterattack.

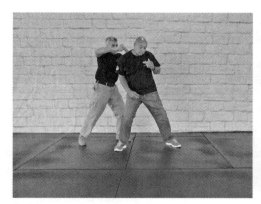 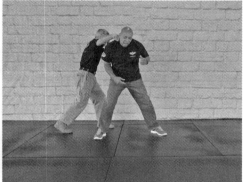

Follow up with a rear straight punch.

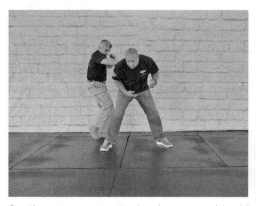 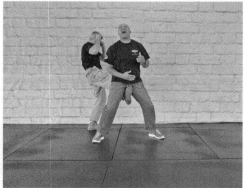

Continue to counterattack using a nearside shin kick to the groin.

Intercepting Side Kick against a Straight Kick

This defense against a low straight kick requires superior timing to intercept the kick with your lead-leg foot.

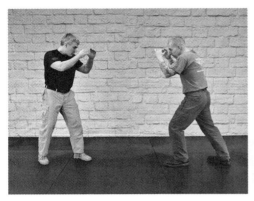 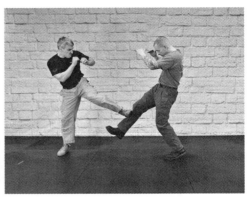

From your regular outlet stance, raise your front leg and turn your foot parallel to the ground, using your foot's entire length, optimally the heel, to intercept your adversary's kicking foot before it has the chance to fully launch. Jam his kick.

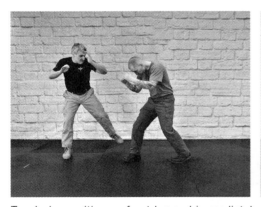 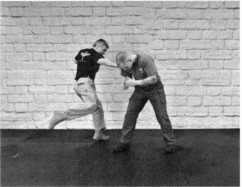

Touch down with your front leg and immediately deliver a strong rear right roundhouse kick.

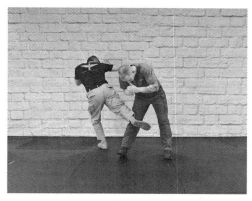

Counterattack immediately as demonstrated by the rear roundhouse shin kick.

Side Kick Defense with Retreat into a Counterkick

One of the best combatives is a low-line side kick. It is difficult to defend. Krav maga uses this kick to cripple an assailant. The same can be done to you. Depending on your retreat and timing, you may absorb the impact on your shin and continue to fight. A good counter is your own counter-side kick, since your leg is raised and chambered in a position to deliver it—the very nature of this defense.

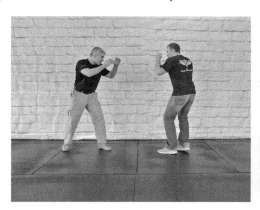
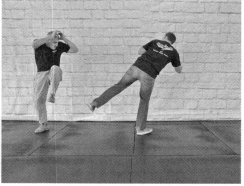

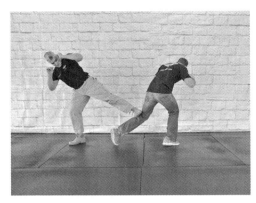

From your left outlet stance, the easiest defense is to raise your targeted leg off the ground and retreat.

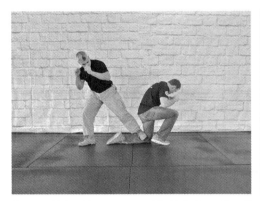 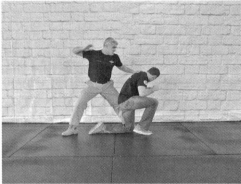

Counterkick with your own side kick, targeting the knee of his incoming leg. The key is not to allow impact to your weight-bearing knee.

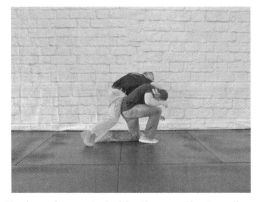

Continue your counterattack as demonstrated by the over-the-top elbow follow-up.

Preemptive Front Kick against a Roundhouse Kick

This defense relies on the principle that the quickest way between two points is a straight line—hence, a straight kick. The defense, therefore, utilizes a straight kick against a low (or any level) rear roundhouse kick targeting the assailant's groin or inside of his thigh or knee as he rolls his hip over to perform the kick. It requires superior timing to preempt the kick with *your* forward leg.

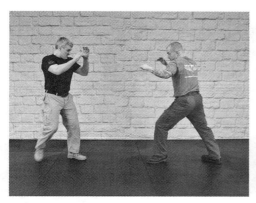 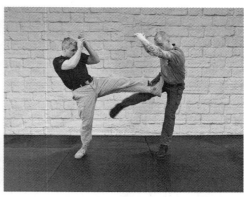

Against any level roundhouse kick, you may deliver a peremptory straight kick to the assailant's groin or thigh, hip, or knee of his kicking leg as he initiates the kick. Follow this with additional retzev combatives. Note: it is also possible, with good timing, to launch a preemptive straight punch to the opponent's throat, jaw, or nose. Remember, however, that leg reach is usually longer than arm reach.

CHAPTER 3

Clinches, Choke and Takedown Defenses, Escorts, and Ground Survival

Close-quarters battle involves different contact ranges best categorized by the distance or proximity as a fight (d)evolves. From a long to medium range, fighters have unfettered movement to batter one another, usually involving long kicks, medium punches, and other hand strikes. From a short range, knees, elbows, head butts, and biting become options. A variety of standing entanglements incorporate medium and short strikes, trapping, clinching, throws, takedowns, and standing joint locks combined for close retzev. The final ground phase occurs when both fighters clinch up in various holds to unbalance and take each other to the ground. This involves medium and short combatives combined with locks and chokes.

Ground movement obviously differs from standing movement. Ground survival can allow one combatant superior control and positioning, preventing the other from defending, disentangling, or escaping as he might while standing. Krav maga groundwork should be thought of as "what you do up, you do down," with additional specific ground-fighting capabilities such as practiced (secondary) weapon deployment for professionals. Remember, krav maga uses many standing combatives on the ground, including groin, eye, and throat strikes in combination with joint breaks and dislocations designed to maim the adversary.

Once engaged against an assailant, the key to most krav maga defenses is a deflection-redirection of the attack combined with a simultaneous body defense and an overwhelming counterattack. Krav maga is designed to stop the attack at its inception or at the earliest possible stage. Closing the distance between the defender and assailant is sometimes referred to as "bursting."

The opposite of bursting is retreating to escape or create distance until an opportunity to close the gap presents itself. As noted, in counterattacking, krav maga usually targets the assailant's soft tissue, including his groin, throat, eyes, and knees. These combatives specifically take into account the adversary's physiological reaction to counterstrikes such as a knee or kick to the groin that will lurch the body forward or a thumb gouge to the eye that will jolt the head back, exposing the groin for further strikes.

If long-range lower-body strikes and intermediate-range upper-body strikes do not neutralize or at least keep your adversary at bay, your adversary can close the distance to grab hold of you. The fight then becomes an "infight" because it involves short combatives, including elbows, knees, uppercut and shovel punches, clinches, and holds. Striking and surprise attacks are integral to clinching and other standing control holds. To strike, you must create separation from your adversary.

Defending against grabs, traps, and takedowns is an indispensable skill. Upper- and lower-body strikes, if improperly executed or well defended by your adversary, can place you in a precarious position resulting in a trap or takedown. Well-executed upper- and lower-body combatives minimize this risk—but there is still a risk, especially if you are fighting against someone who is skilled in ground combat.

Clinching can broadly be thought of as any control grasp on an adversary's body while both adversaries are still standing. Clinching can also involve compact, powerful strikes and control holds when two adversaries are standing in close proximity to one another. Certain types of clinches are also referred to in defensive krav maga vernacular as "bear hugs."

In this chapter you'll learn many infighting techniques and defenses. They all rely on the same principles: always fight back by attacking the weakest points of your adversary's anatomy and by using his momentum against him. Once your assailant closes on you, he can attempt life-threatening choke holds, throws, strikes, and neck manipulations. Other types of close-contact grappling include hair pulling, headlocks, and bear hugs, all of which can put you into an extremely exposed position.

Striking in a clinch is different from striking from a distance. In a clinch, body contact can be used to control your adversary. This is especially relevant when an adversary goes to the ground and no longer has the upright support of his legs. Therefore, body contact dictates your fight strategy. In fighting, it is common for one or both adversaries to lose balance, either as a result of tactics or chance, so you need to be prepared for that possibility.

Off-balancing is key to close-quarters infighting. The objective is to take your adversary off balance by setting up retzev combatives including strikes, throws, and joint locks. Wherever the head goes, the body will follow. Taking an adversary off balance allows you to set up other retzev combative techniques because the adversary is not only concerned with protecting himself but with recovering his balance. Take the adversary in a direction he does not expect to go. Space restraints do not allow us to illustrate the all-important retzev or continuous combat follow-through; however, we have included a few techniques and shown partial retzev to give you adequate insight into combined defense and attack through continuous combat motion.

Clinching

In a superior clinch position, you can trap your opponent's head and torso, making both defense and counterattack difficult for him while maintaining your own combative options—primarily, elbows, short punches, uppercuts, hooks, shovel punches, knee strikes to the groin and midsection (especially switching knees and roundhouse knee shots), locks, chokes, takedowns, and throws. (Clinches are also used for military tactics that are not depicted here for security concerns.) You may, of course, also gouge your adversary's eyes with your thumbs prior to acquiring control of the head. You must be aware, however, that an adversary could deploy a weapon to attack you while both of your hands are occupied with controlling his head. The clinch can give you several advantages by controlling

1. your adversary's ability to strike you,
2. your position for powerful, short, devastating combatives, and
3. his attempts to take you down.

The last point requires emphasis. The clinch can both save you from being taken down and can allow you to take your adversary down, depending on how you use it.

We will focus primarily on the crown-of-the-head and rear clinches, which afford great control over your adversary. These clinches provide the option of strikes and takedowns into superior ground-fighting positions. A third clinching position heavily emphasized in the krav maga curriculum is the symmetrical clinch because it is frequently used.

Crown-of-the-Head Clinch

This powerful hold allows you strong control of your adversary by clasping the crown of his skull, setting you up to perform knee strikes, vertical-elbows guillotine chokes, and neck-torquing movements. You may also gouge his eyes with your thumb prior to encircling his head with your arms. Always vie for inside hand position to allow better control over the adversary. Inside hand position means both of your arms are inside your adversary's arms and exerting pressure on the rear crown of his head. If you control the head, you can usually control the body. Try not to grab the base of the neck because the opponent can better resist the hold. Do not interlock you fingers in this (or any other) hold because your fingers can be broken and the opponent can more readily control your hands.

In addition, the crown-of-the head clinch is highly useful for transitioning to military terminal-force applications.

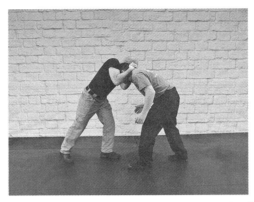

Place one hand on the crown of your adversary's head and your other hand on top of the first. Squeeze your elbows together, forcing your adversary's head to your chest level to further off-balance him. Do not secure him by his neck. Keep your adversary's head lower than your own and pressed into your chest.

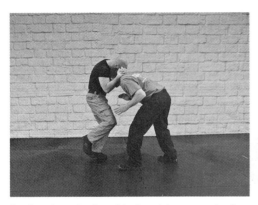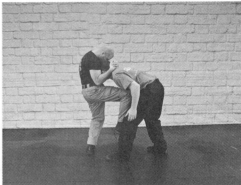

Again, do not allow his head to separate from your chest. To defend this type of clinch, you might target the groin and the eye socket—so, your adversary might do the same to you. This is one of the drawbacks of this technique.

Clinch Defense

The clinch can place you in a position susceptible to devastating knees, elbows, and neck manipulations. A simple defense is to keep one elbow close to your body and pointed downward to defend against knees while using your other hand to attack your adversary's eyes with a thumb gouge or eye rake.

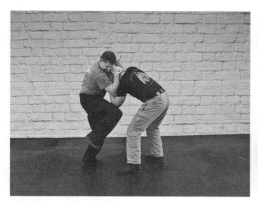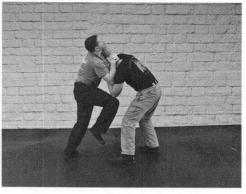

Keep one elbow down, using the tip to defend against knee strikes. Simultaneously access his eye socket even if he buries his head. Another defense is to yank down on one arm keeping your elbow tip down, positioned to defend against knee strikes.

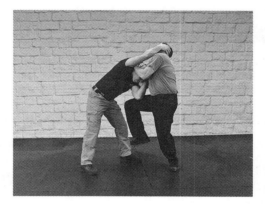

Tackle Defenses

You must be able to defend against an adversary changing his level of attack. Combatants often set up successful takedowns using a distraction (usually an upper-body strike feint). While the combative distraction may or may not connect, it will allow him to lower his level and close on you to secure your legs.

Note: the following defenses assume the defender did not have time or the opportunity to deliver a straight kick or knee to the head, or to sidestep the takedown using a jam to the head or combatives.

Inline Sprawl

When defending against a tackle or two-leg takedown, if timing and distance do not allow a combative, evasive sidestep, or both, you may use an "inline" sprawl. Sprawl backward using one arm as the "brake" to prevent the assailant from taking you down or securing your legs.

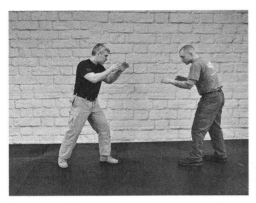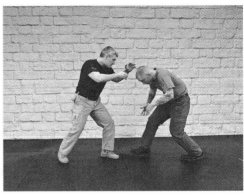

From your left outlet stance, as the assailant lowers his height to attempt the takedown, lower your level while dropping your right arm as you sidestep to intercept the assailant on his left trapezius muscle.

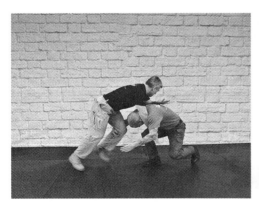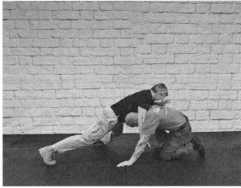

Sprawl on the balls of your feet while shooting your legs back and wide for a stable platform—but not so wide that you cannot comfortably rest on the balls of your feet.

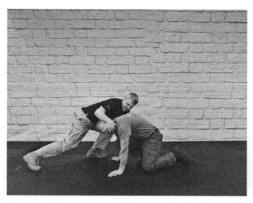 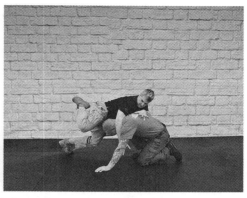

As you drop down with the assailant, immediately knee him in the head to jolt the spine, rip his eyes, or use a north-south position to choke him.

Offline Sprawl

When defending against a tackle, if timing and distance do not allow a combative, you may use an offline sprawl where you stay on your feet to get up immediately and stomp the assailant's head.

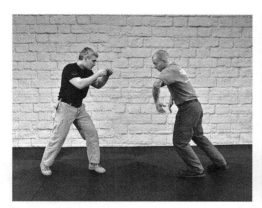 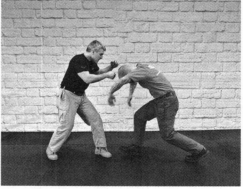

From your left outlet stance, as the assailant lowers his height to attempt the takedown, side-step slightly to enable your right arm to shoot down, intercepting the assailant on his right trapezius muscle.

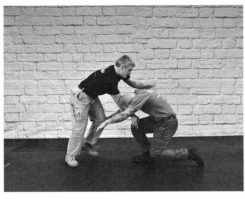 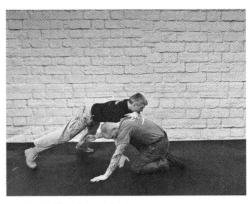

Shoot your legs back wide for a stable platform on the balls of your feet.

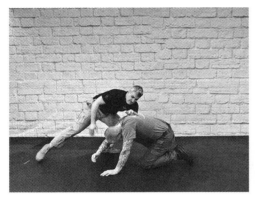 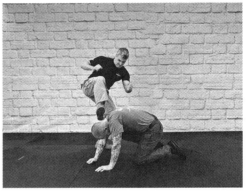

If you go down with the assailant, you can immediately knee him in the head to jolt the spine. Stand up immediately to deliver a heel kick to the assailant's neck or head.

Release from a Standing Professional Blood Choke

This attack must be defended immediately. It is crucial that you clamp down on the assailant's arm, using your core strength to exert counterpressure. If the adversary is using a figure-four or "professional choke" grip, you must yank down on the crook of the assailant's elbow while clearing the other hand from behind your head.

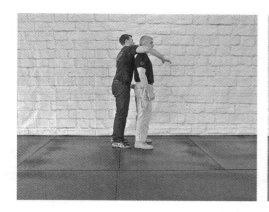
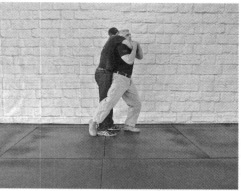

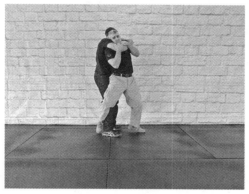

Tuck your chin while grabbing the assailant's forearm and biceps muscle with each of your hands. Use your core, not just your upper body, to yank down, applying counterpressure against the assailant's choking arm.

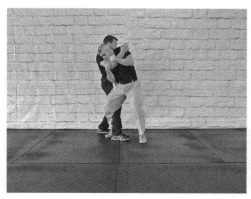
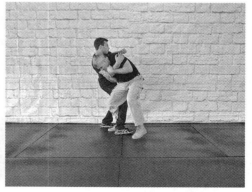

Maintain strong counterpressure and continue to turn into the assailant's choking arm. Simultaneously step around the assailant's nearside leg (the same leg as his choking arm side) to take him down. As you turn into the assailant, simultaneously begin to trip him by catching his leg with your leg while forcing him to his rear nearside corner. You also have the option of sweeping the assailant's leg as you force his upper body backward.

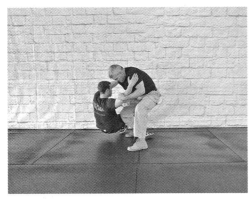 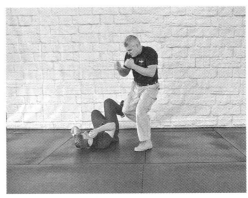

As you apply counterpressure, take a decisive step outside while maintaining contact with the assailant's same-side leg. You must "marry" your leg to his. If you have separation, he could defeat the defense and continue to choke you.

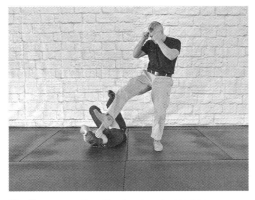

Continue counterattacks as necessary.

Release from a Standing Professional Blood Choke, Variation

Once again, this attack must be defended immediately. It is crucial that you clamp down on the assailant's arms using your core strength. This defense may be used if you errantly turn *in the direction of the choke* (the opposite direction of the previous defense). Use your core, not just your upper body, to yank down and apply counterpressure on the assailant's choking arm and his hand clutching his own biceps.

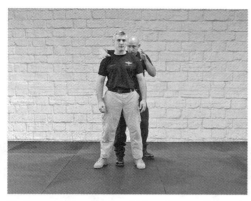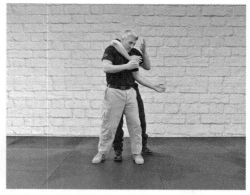

Tuck your chin while grabbing the assailant's forearm and his opposite arm's biceps muscle with each of your respective arms.

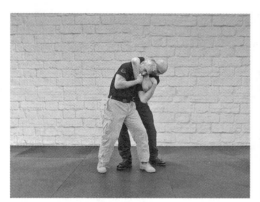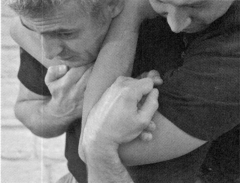

As you maintain steady counterpressure, continue to turn into the assailant's choking arm and forcibly strip his hand from his biceps by getting the strongest grip on his fingers. Note the close-up of the hand strip.

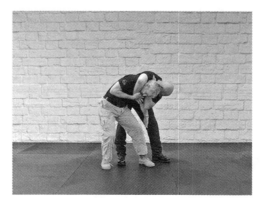

After you momentarily relieve pressure from the choke by stripping the assailant's hand, continue to apply counterpressure with both arms. As soon as the hand is stripped, move slightly to the side (defender's right in the photo) to expose the assailant's groin to hand strikes.

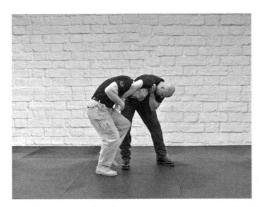 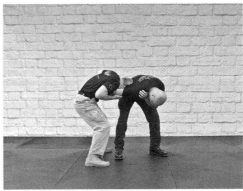

Continue to maintain counterpressure against the forearm as you counterattack and slip your head out of his hold. Be aware that your gear or webbing may impede your stepping back and underneath the hold to release.

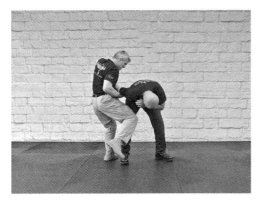 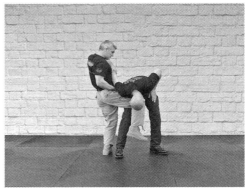

After you force the assailant to release the tight choke, maintain contact and pressure with his forward arm. As you create an opening, take a slight step back with your inside leg (nearside leg in relation to the assailant). Maintain contact with his choking arm against your torso as you step out to release the choke. Continue to keep the arm pinned and deliver devastating knee counter-attacks to neutralize the threat. Control #6 from this position is a good takedown for those who need to apply restraints.

Rear Naked Choke Defense Driven Forward into Seoi Nage Drop

These techniques allow the defender to naturally move forward with the forward choking pressure to counterattack by executing a strong throw. The *seoi nage* drop against a rear choke driving you forward requires you to slightly offset your hips from the assailant's hips. The drop allows you to throw your assailant by sinking your hips lower than his to jettison him from your back. Note: gear and webbing may create space or "slack" between your torso and the attacker's torso. Overcome any artificial space by securing his body as tightly to your torso as you can when you launch him. Note: this technique may also be performed with a double knee drop.

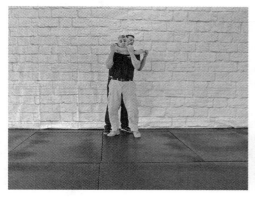 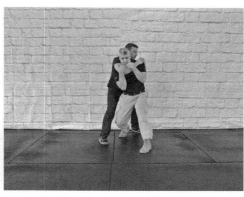

Yank down on the assailant's choking arm (in this case the crook of the elbow) while tucking your chin. The adversary's choking arm serves as a handle to launch him.

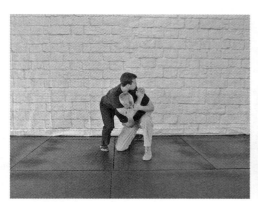 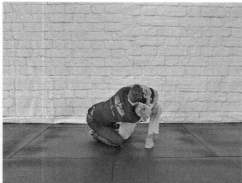

As the assailant drives you forward, drop to your inside knee while forcibly locking down on the choking arm. Whip your upper body slightly to the left (as depicted in the photo) to launch the assailant to the right corner.

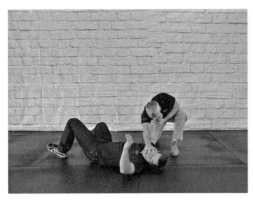 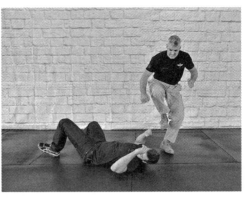

The moment you complete the throw, follow with retzev such as an eye gouge or kick to the head (only if necessary). If you fall with the assailant, be sure to drop your weight on him to both increase his impact with the ground and to save yourself from striking the ground.

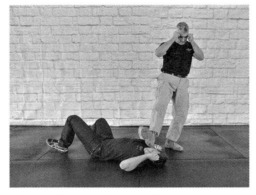

If necessary, finish the defense with a heel kick or other combative.

Defensive Throw against an Assailant Jumping onto the Defender's Back

Similar to the previous technique, this tactic allows the defender to naturally move forward with the forward choking pressure to counterattack by executing a strong throw. This hip toss defense to counter a rear choke driving you forward requires you to square or slightly offset your hips from the assailant's hips. Use both the assailant's forward momentum and your forward momentum against him.

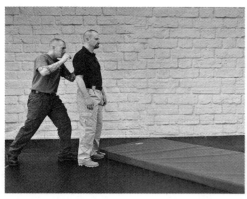 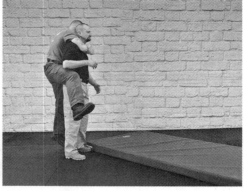

Defend against a rear jumping headlock or choke by plucking or yanking down on the assailant's arms while tucking your chin. The assailant's choking arm serves as a handle to throw him. If the attacker hooks his left leg, use your left hand to thwart this attempt by peeling the top of his foot or heel while continuing to defend the choke with your right as you launch him.

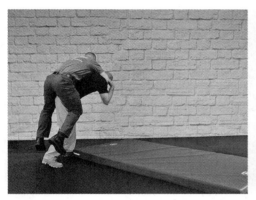 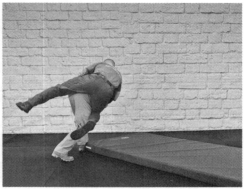

Lock down on the assailant's arm as you move forward with the momentum of the attack. Bend both of your legs slightly while turning your body to the side.

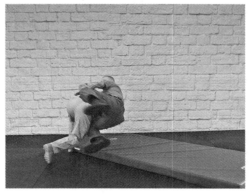

The moment you complete the throw, follow with retzev. If you fall with the assailant, be sure to drop your weight on him to both increase his impact with the ground and save yourself from impacting the ground.

Defensive Throw against a Rear Choke When the Assailant Is Pulling the Defender Backward (Osoto Makikomi Variation)

This is an extremely difficult attack to defend, as the assailant has created torso separation and is pulling you backward, undermining your base. The key to the defense is to proceed (as learned previously) with your upper-body counterpressure; however, to defeat this attack you must work with your left far-side leg by raising it in the air to generate momentum to throw him.

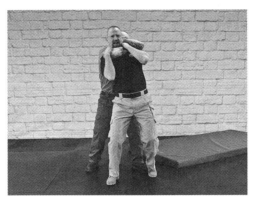

As the assailant ratchets up the pressure, pulling you backward, tuck your chin and latch on to his choking arm, using your core strength to resist the choke.

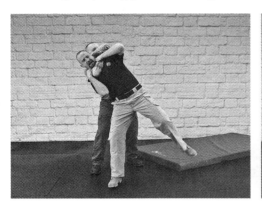
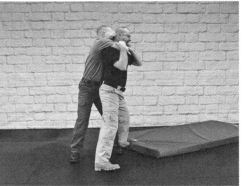

As you resist the choke, shoot your left far-side leg straight up and then sweep it backward to land on one or both of your knees. Lifting the leg is crucial to facilitate the torque you will need to throw the assailant forcefully over your back.

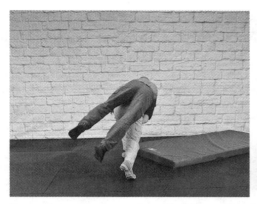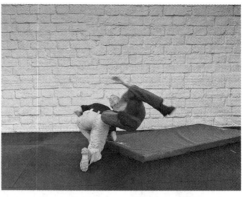

Depending on your core strength, it is possible for you to land all of your weight on your assailant by landing on the balls of your feet instead of your knees.

Escort Control Holds

Krav maga employs eight different escort control holds designed to move a prisoner or control a belligerent person. Anyone who has had to control or restrain a determined resisting subject ("controlee") understands the difficulty of applying minimum use-of-force controls. Accordingly, krav maga advocates using a "softener" combative or series of combatives targeting the "green" zones or anatomical targets that, when struck, will not result in long-term physical damage or death.

The control holds switch from one control tactic to another when a person resists. The switch is a form of retzev. These holds can be applied by one or two escorting or controlling officers, agents, or security personnel. Part of our specific focus in krav maga is to allow multiple responding personnel to subdue a person quickly and efficiently without placing pressure or force against a controlee's spine, base of the neck, or throat. I have elected to cover escort control holds #2, #3, #4, #6, and #7. I have omitted escort control holds #1 and #5, as these are somewhat height dependent and not suitable for all practitioners.

Krav maga also has countermeasures to its own control holds; however, once again with the goals of this book in mind, these are not depicted but reserved for vetted, in-person training. In learning the countermeasures to our own control holds, our trainees become more efficient in administering the control holds.

Standing Escort Control Holds #6 and #7 may also be used to take a hostile third party swiftly and efficiently to the ground to apply restraints, to wait for additional help, or to de-escalate a situation. These takedown holds are thoroughly covered in *Krav Maga Weapon Defenses* (YMAA, 2012), chapter 1.

Control #2

Control #2 is designed to restrain a standing controlee's freedom of movement while allowing the controller to escort him or her to a different location.

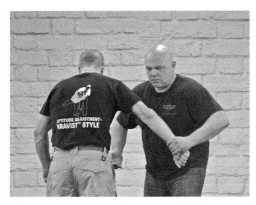 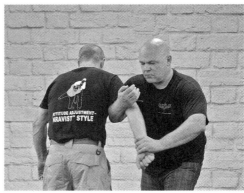

With your left arm, seize control of the controlee's right arm by his right wrist. Note: it is also possible to secure the controlee's arm by securing the back of the controlee's hand. As you seize control, drive the top of your right forearm (radial bone) into the controlee's elbow joint, forcing the controlee to bend his elbow.

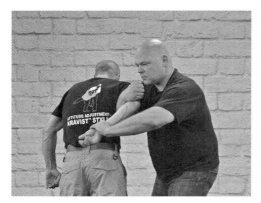 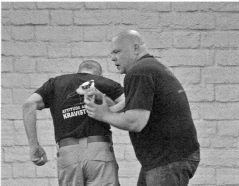

As you force the controlee's arm to bend, use your torso and body mass to place the controlee's arm against his body with your right arm interlaced between the controlee's arm and the controlee's body. Do not allow any space between your torso and the controlee's arm. Once you have forced the controlee's arm back and slightly away, seize the controlee's hand, forcing it also back and away to apply a wristlock.

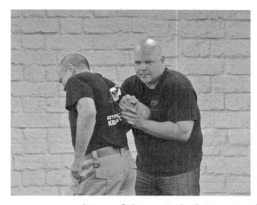

Once the wristlock is secure, you may let go of the controlee's arm to seize the controlee's wrist with both hands. Or you can administer a combination hold by reaching around to the controlee's face to force the controlee's nose, applying pressure at the philtrum, up and away to facilitate the escort while using de-escalation language to make the controlee more cooperative. Instead of the philtrum, you can also use his eye socket.

Control #3

Control Hold #3 is designed to restrain a standing controlee's freedom of movement while allowing the controller to escort him or her to a different location or to force the controlee to the ground for additional restraints or de-escalatory tactics. By design, Control #3 flows from Control #2.

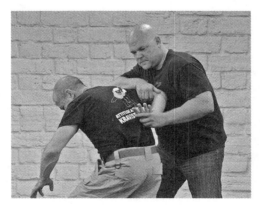

Similar to Control #2, with your left arm seize control of your adversary's right arm. Grasp his right wrist by the back of the hand, forcing his arm toward his torso. Note: it is also possible to secure his arm by securing the back of his hand. As you force the controlee's targeted arm to bend, use your torso and body mass to place his arm against his body with your right arm and hand clamping down on his inner triceps, just above the elbow. Do not allow any space between your torso and the controlee's arm. Once you have forced his arm back and slightly away, if you are more physically powerful than the controlee or, perhaps, evenly matched with him and you can seize the initiative, you can force his arm and shoulder up and away, creating significant pressure to make him stoop forward. You may now escort the controlee away while using de-escalation language to make him more cooperative. If you feel it is necessary to take him to the ground, you can place greater pressure on his arm and shoulder, forcing him forward in a two o'clock position, or at about a 30-degree angle. Forcing the controlee forward at this angle prevents him from rolling on his side to undermine the control hold.

Control #4

Control #4 is designed to restrain a standing controlee's freedom of movement while allowing the controller to escort him or her to a different location. By design, Control #4 flows from Controls #2 and #3 if the controlee resists and pulls his or her arm forward.

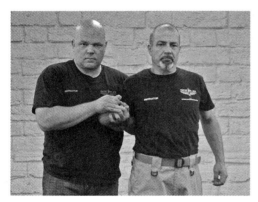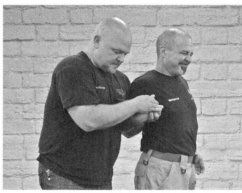

Seize control of your adversary's right wrist with your left hand as you drive your right forearm into his elbow joint, forcing him to bend his elbow. He will likely pull back in resistance. Corral his momentum by securing his wrist, forcing his elbow and triceps muscle back toward your torso. Interlace your right arm between the controlee's arm and his body. Do not allow any space between your torso and his arm. Once the wristlock is secure, you may let go of his arm with your left arm to seize his wrist with both hands. Or you can administer a combination hold by reaching around to the controlee's face to force his nose (philtrum) up and away, facilitating . the escort while using de-escalation language to make him more cooperative.

Control #6

Control #6 allows you to swiftly take down a controlee, driving him into the ground face first and achieving strong deadside positional control, as well as dominant control over any weapon. The hold places compliance or takedown pressure on the controlee's wrist and shoulder while securing the controlee's arm. Control #6 may be applied with or without preceding retzev combatives. An accompanying lower-body combative forces the controlee's level down to facilitate Control #6. This control is designed to restrain a standing controlee's freedom of movement while allowing the controller to escort him or her to a different location or force the controlee to the ground for additional restraints or de-escalatory tactics. (Also see pages 12–14 of *Krav Maga Weapon Defenses* [YMAA, 2012] for additional photos of Control #6 [otherwise referred to as Control Hold "A"].)

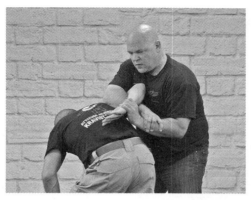

Seize control of your adversary's right arm by his right wrist. Seizing the arm is usually accompanied by a lower-body combative to the green zone, such as a straight knee strike to the thigh or kick to the shin. After administering combatives, grab his right wrist with your left hand. Note: it is also possible to secure the controlee's arm by securing the back of his hand. Use the radial bone (top of the forearm) of your right arm to knife through at the controlee's elbow, forcing him to bend his arm. Raise your wrist to place upward pressure so his arm comes up with a 90-degree bend with fingers toward the ground. Reach over the top of his targeted shoulder, clamping down hard on the shoulder while snaking your right arm over the top of his right arm and across his shoulder to clasp your other arm. You must clamp down on the targeted shoulder to facilitate the lock. Reach around the arm and encircle it to grip your own forearm. Bring his elbow and wrist close to your body, torquing the shoulder upward while keeping hard pressure on the shoulder. Place considerable pressure on the shoulder by wrenching up and away while keeping the controlee's torso flush with yours to force him forward in a two o'clock position, or about a 30-degree angle. Forcing the controlee forward at this particular angle prevents him from rolling on his side, thereby undermining Control #6.

Note: by torquing the arm upward, an escape—especially using a scissors takedown or counter—becomes much more difficult. Take a 180-degree (tai-sabaki) step toward two o'clock with your right leg to bring down your opponent. As your opponent is going down, keep the grip tight. You may further secure him and the weapon by placing your right knee behind his elbow, exerting pressure up on the shoulder, and your left knee on top of his neck. Remove any weapon by peeling it from the assailant's grip, using your thumb at the grip's base to keep the point directed at him and away from you.

Control #7

Control #7 allows an assailant to be taken swiftly backward and down with strong deadside control. This hold can be administered if the controlee has an edged weapon in his hand. Control #7 may be applied with or without preceding retzev combatives. Usually, the defender has delivered strong preceding combatives and has control of the weapon arm before applying the specific hold. The hold places compliance or takedown pressure on the opponent's shoulder and wrist while controlling the weapon. (See also pages 15–17 of *Krav Maga Weapon Defenses* [YMAA, 2012] for additional photos of Control Hold #7 [otherwise referred to as Control Hold "B"].)

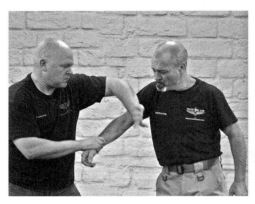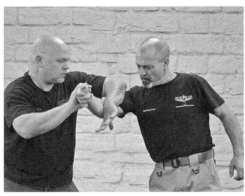

If you are facing or positioned to the side of your opponent, secure his right wrist with your left hand. Grip the flat of the back of his hand with a perpendicular grip. You can push his face away to cause a distraction. Curl his wrist in while slipping your other arm on the shoulder over the top of his targeted arm and across his forearm, using a figure-four grip.

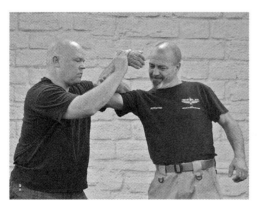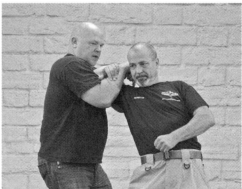

Reach around the arm and encircle it to grip your own forearm, tightening your right arm to your body. Bring his elbow and wrist close to your body while keeping the grip tight.

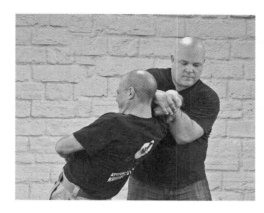

For law enforcement and security personnel, or others who may wish to exert maximum control of the assailant, when effecting the hold against a perpetrator, armed or unarmed, once you have taken the opponent down on his back, you may reverse him onto his stomach. Yank up on his arm while still maintaining your figure-four grip, and then turn in the opposite direction. Do not break the movements by touching your knees to the ground. Be sure not to collapse with him, and keep upward pressure on his arm as you rotate him. Maintain the momentum of the takedown into an immediate reversal onto his stomach.

By keeping strong pressure on his wrist and shoulder to facilitate his turn, you have taken him down by combining a joint lock and a 180-degree step in one direction. Now take a 180-degree (tai-sabaki) step in the opposite direction. This second opposite turn begins to turn him onto his stomach. (See *Krav Maga Weapon Defenses* [YMAA, 2012], pages 15–17 for additional photos.) When employing this technique against an armed assailant, remove the weapon by peeling it from his grip, using your thumb at the grip's base to keep the point directed at him and away from you. You are now in a strong position to remove the weapon, apply restraints, and control his movement. Once you have forced the controlee's arm back and slightly away, seize the controlee's hand, forcing it back and away into a wristlock.

Core Ground Survival Tactics

Beginning in the early 1990s, Grandmaster Haim Gidon began to revamp the krav maga curriculum, adding extensive ground survival tactics approved by Imi, who sat in Haim's gym, monitoring, mentoring, and enjoying the continuing evolution of krav maga. What follows are some of the fruits of Haim's dedication to improving krav maga.

As noted earlier, Israeli krav maga ground survival can generally be summarized, "What we do up, we do down." In other words, whatever we do from an upright position, with modification and your weight properly positioned, we do from a ground position. This includes positioning the defender for optimum secondary-weapon deployment. And just as there are no rules in an "up" fight, there are no rules in a "down" fight. Groin strikes, throat strikes, eye gouges, and biting are all viable and are ground fighting options.

Do not go to the ground if it can be helped. A second assailant or multiple assailants could come to the first assailant's aid. To state the obvious, fighting multiple adversaries on the ground is extremely difficult—hence the importance of developing your infighting and anti-takedown capabilities to remain standing.

Krav maga ground techniques incorporate both defensive and offensive tactics. In this book, we will only examine a few of the core techniques involving the most common ground survival situations.

Professional krav maga training also takes into account limitations that may be imposed on the defender's movements and flexibility due to equipment, such as a duty belt, bulletproof vest, flak jacket, or backpack. It's relatively easy to execute triangle chokes and other complex techniques in a dojo; on the street or in a combat zone, while wearing heavy equipment, it is much more difficult. Practical hindrances such as trying to apply an Achilles leg lock to an assailant wearing high rigid combat boots must also be taken into account when learning professional krav maga tactics.

Foreleg Brace Position (Modified "Z Guard")

The "brakes" technique uses a horizontal knee brace to disengage you from an assailant who is trying to mount you or spread your legs. By turning on your side (which may also be used as a weapon-retention tactic until it is opportune to deploy a sidearm or edged weapon), raise one leg to use your shin and knee to keep an assailant at bay as you deliver combatives such as eye gouges, throat strikes, punches, and knee strikes. Your hips and legs are your most powerful muscle groups.

As you separate yourself from your assailant, forcefully extend your foreleg to both strike and push away from your opponent. You will likely gain the opportunity to kick him in the groin or head, using a straight kick or side kick while on the ground, both delivered with the heel. Make contact with your heel to the groin, midsection, or face. Get up immediately by sliding your underneath leg back and onto the ball of your foot while posting one hand on the ground and keeping one hand up to deliver more combatives and make your escape.

Foreleg Brace ("Z Guard") Transitioning to a Handgun

The key to deploying a secondary weapon, in this case a handgun, is to create enough separation to be able to withdraw the handgun, get a clean line of fire (with none of your body parts in front of the muzzle), and squeeze the trigger as necessary. Crucially, the handgun must only be deployed when the defender is in a position to shoot. In other words, the assailant must not have an opportunity to disarm the defender or seize the weapon.

Legs play a crucial role in creating the necessary space. To push the assailant away to separation, krav maga's preferred position on the ground is the foreleg brace position, or inserting the defender's legs using one foreleg and the heel of the opposite leg.

Generally, the system does not embrace the guard because the groin is susceptible to attack including punches, elbow strikes, grabs, head butts, and biting. (Note: there are two positions in which the system does emphasize the guard: wrenching the neck and the seated guillotine.)

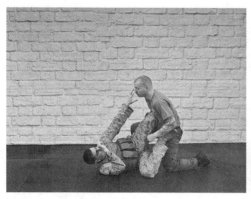 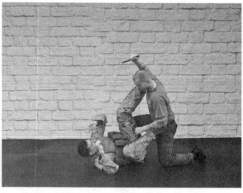

Roll onto your right hip and insert the shin and patella of your top leg against the assailant's lower torso. Simultaneously insert your lower heel against the assailant's hip or thigh. You may use your top leg to stop an incoming attack as depicted.

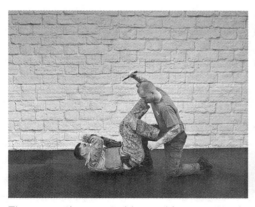 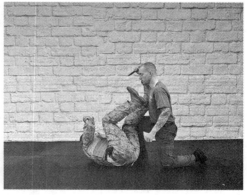

The separation created by pushing your two legs together (foreleg and opposite heel) will allow you to administer a strong heel kick to the face, throat, or solar plexus with your bottom-side leg.

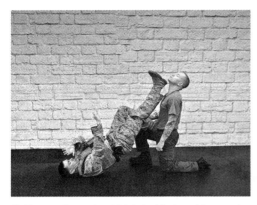 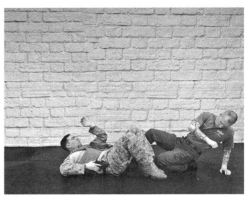

Deliver a strong heel kick to his head to create separation, enabling you to deploy your sidearm.

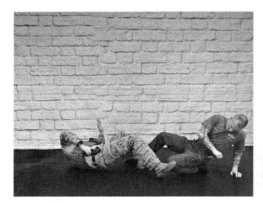 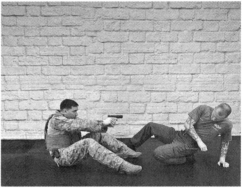

Use a modified shrimp or side shimmy to push yourself further away from the assailant while deploying your sidearm. Immediately position the handgun between your legs for a stable and accurate firing platform. Be sure to keep your legs down and away from the line of fire. It is possible to turn one foot parallel to the ground, toes facing the side (not toes up), to provide a kick option to create separation.

Foreleg Brace into Armbar

The foreleg brace also allows transitions into armbars (and triangle chokes, the next technique presented). Remember, the preference is to create separation and damage to the opponent with kicks, and get right to your feet. Again, being on the ground is dangerous for the myriad of reasons previously discussed. Nevertheless, ground survival by necessity incorporates maiming or strangling an opponent. This defense is a modification of a standing technique covered in chapter 2, Sliding Parry While Stepping Off the Line.

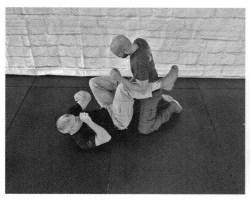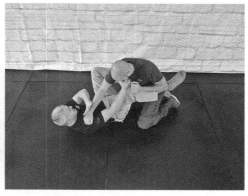

From the foreleg brace position, parry the punch by deflecting and sliding up the assailant's right incoming arm with your left arm while simultaneously attacking his eyes with a finger strike (making sure to keep your fingers bent to avoid damaging them).

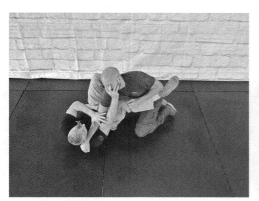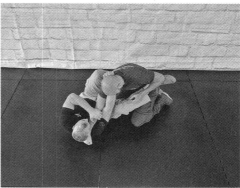

Secure the assailant's outstretched arm by clamping down on it while using your striking hand to secure him at the trapezius, grabbing his shirt to prevent him from retracting his arm.

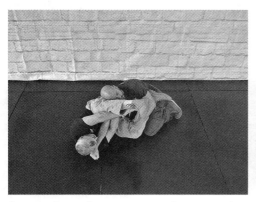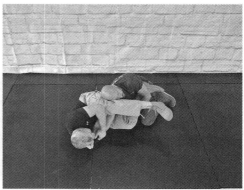

As you clamp down to secure the targeted arm, swing your left leg in front of the assailant's face. Yank back forcefully on his right arm to extend it as much as possible as you extend your left leg across his face.

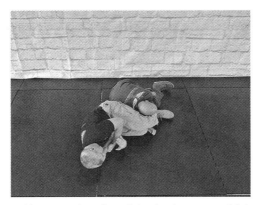

Secure the arm tightly, making sure the elbow joint is above your thighs, and extend your body back as you use your core strength to dislocate the elbow joint.

Foreleg Brace into Short Triangle Choke

The foreleg brace also allows transitions into triangle choke holds. Again, the best-case scenario is to create space, damage with kicks, and get to your feet. Surviving on the ground sometimes means maiming or strangling the enemy.

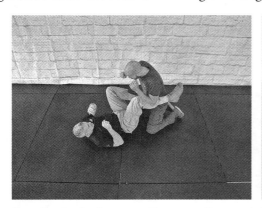
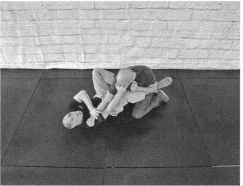

From the foreleg brace position, parry the punch by deflecting and sliding up the assailant's right incoming arm with your left arm while simultaneously attacking his eyes with a fingers strike. Be sure to keep your fingers bent to avoid damaging them.

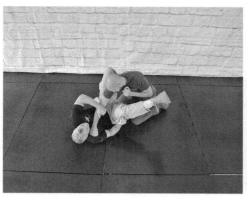
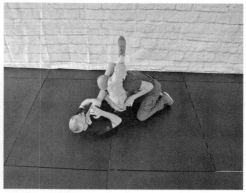

Secure the assailant's outstretched arm by forcefully clamping down on it while swinging your bottom right leg over his left shoulder. Then wrap your right leg around his shoulder.

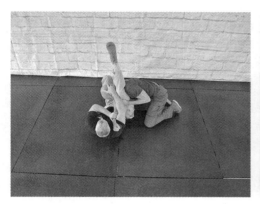
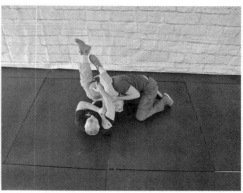

As you clamp down on his head and shoulders, raise your left leg up slightly to insert your right ankle in the crook of your left knee to create the triangle choke by restricting blood flow on both sides of his neck.

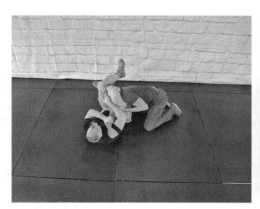
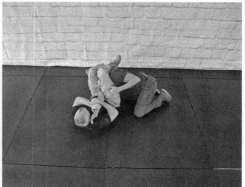

Squeeze your right leg down into his head while simultaneously clamping down on your right leg with your left leg to optimize the human vice. Pull his head toward you with your right arm to further increase the choking pressure.

Inside Knee While Attacking the Eyes

If you are unable to obtain the foreleg brace position, the next best position is inserting your nearside knee to keep the assailant from mounting you. Then create separation and deploy a weapon, as necessary.

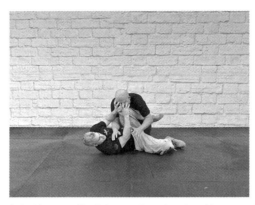

Pull your nearside knee into the assailant to create a barrier. Use your fingers to rake his eyes to facilitate separation to allow additional kicks, secondary weapon deployment, and to get up off the ground.

Protecting Your Neck

Protecting your head, neck, and spine during a confrontation is vital. The ability to defend against chokes and neck manipulations is paramount in all aspects of a fight, particularly in a ground scenario. A broken neck or spine can paralyze or kill. Hair may be used to torque the neck, exposing the throat to attack. (To yank the head back, you need to grasp the front of the scalp, running your fingers through the hair and making a tight fist to increase the leverage of the pull.) Having closely cropped hair or no hair provides an advantage to guard against such neck manipulations.

Counterattacks to the head and neck can shut the body down temporarily or permanently. The neck is extremely vulnerable because of its vital air passages, arteries, and nerves that sustain proper brain function. The spinal column is highly susceptible to injury at the base of the neck from strikes, throws, and locks, with potentially lethal consequences if the spinal nerves are severed. Striking, manipulating, and twisting the neck can injure the arteries and vertebrae. In a defensive mode, you must take great care to protect these vital areas through proper technique and body positioning. Chokes are quick fight enders. Obviously, you must not allow anyone to get his hands, arms, or legs around your neck.

Techniques that force the head forward, back, or sideways can produce serious injury to the neck, specifically the cervical vertebrae. The key to executing proper chokes is using your hands and arms to provide leverage and compression against an adversary's throat and neck, leaving him few, if any, defenses. The narrower the choking implement, the easier the penetration to the adversary's neck. The ulnar and radial edges of the wrist and forearm are particularly well suited to apply compression to the throat and neck.

Defending the Mount

If an adversary were to successfully mount you, he could rain down a hail of strikes while pinning you to the ground. Gravity works for him and against you. Similar to most krav maga defenses, you need to attack his vulnerable anatomy—in this case, the groin. As you attack the groin, simultaneously buck him off you.

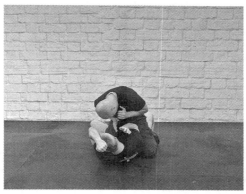

Counterattack his groin using a short elbow strike.

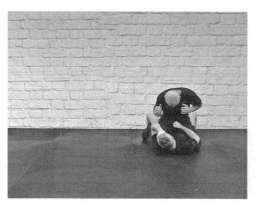
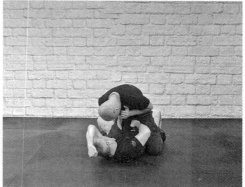

Another option is to deliver a hammer fist to the groin while keeping your other hand up to protect your head. A third option is to deliver a downward straight punch, again keeping your cover hand up.

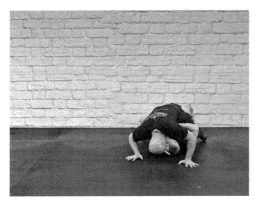 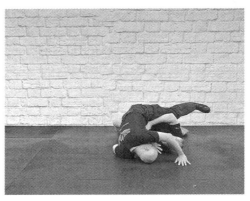

As you deliver the strike to the groin, buck the adversary to the *opposite corner* of the strike. In other words, the defender strikes with his right arm and propels the assailant at an approximate 45-degree angle to his left (the assailant's right).

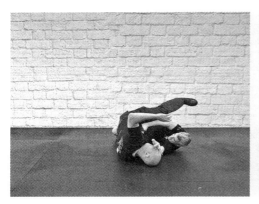 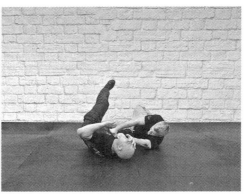

Continue to throw the adversary to the designated corner using your upper body in concert with your hip buck. Continue your counterattacks, including eye strikes and additional combatives to the groin. Get up immediately.

Protecting the Throat and Neck

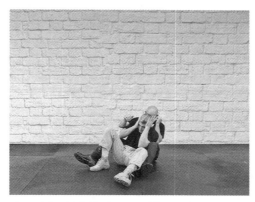

Protecting your throat and neck is vital. Tuck your chin and keep your shoulders shrugged as an initial defense against an attack to the neck; however, these are only preliminary measures and you must reverse the position immediately.

These preliminary defenses can easily be defeated by an assailant who yanks your hair back or applies pressure against your philtrum, eye sockets, or other pressure points. Professional krav maga focuses on just a few proven neck breaks and strangleholds. It is not appropriate to show these tactics here.

Deadside and Positional Control Strategy Revisited

Once committed to a fight, put yourself in a dominant position. Never turn your back to your adversary in any type of fight situation, especially if this puts you facedown on the ground, the worst possible position. From this position the back of your head and neck are exposed to attack. Nearly as dangerous is if the adversary secures you from behind or "takes your back" with his legs hooked around your torso or employs a body triangle clamp where he folds one leg under a knee, creating a figure four. As with deadside position in a standing fight, optimally you will achieve a side-mount or rear-mount position in a ground fight. There are four preferred krav maga ground positions: rear mount, side straddle, side mount with chest down, and the high mount while controlling the adversary's arms. Punishing combatives, joint-break locks, and choke options are readily available from these positions.

Krav maga rarely relies on joint-lock breaks and chokes without first engaging in retzev combative attacks. Think of it as softening up your adversary. An adversary defending against combative strikes may put himself in a vulnerable position for joint-break locks and chokes. Many fighters rely heavily on the hands for combatives and the feet primarily for movement. Keep in mind that in a ground fight the legs become highly important for gaining control over an adversary. To achieve a lock, it is paramount that you keep your hips close to your adversary's targeted joint. Positional control is crucial. Ease of transition or ground retzev must be second nature.

A Note on the Mount and High Closed-Guard Positions

The mount (where you are straddling your adversary with his back to the ground and your heels are hooked underneath his ribcage) and the high closed guard (where your back is to the ground and your adversary is pincered between your legs, which are hooked at the ankles) are well-known and formidable fighting positions. There should be little doubt of their proven efficacy in the ring. Yet there is one crucial street-fighting vulnerability if your adversary maintains proper position: your groin, throat, and eyes are also susceptible to attack.

Note that the best release and defense against locks, either while standing or on the ground, is to avoid putting yourself in a vulnerable position in the first place. As noted, chokes and joint-lock breaks are fight enders. While you can use them with great efficiency, remember they can be used against you. Keeping your chin tucked and limbs safe is key. This preemptive body positioning cannot be overemphasized.

Rear Naked Choke Defense (Warding Off the Hooks)

When fighting on the ground, if an assailant takes your back, you are in grave danger that he will apply a choke. He can also rake your eyes and pummel your head. A good ground fighter will pincer his legs around you to prevent your escape, and extend his body by stretching his legs and upper body in opposite directions to strengthen the choke or face bar. You are also in jeopardy of the assailant delivering punishing heel kicks to your groin (as you might do to an adversary).

A choke from the rear mount is one of the worst positions you can find yourself in, but it is not indefensible. However, it must be defended immediately before the adversary can sink the choke and hook his legs around you. Biting the assailant's forearm is an effective option to facilitate the release.

Your objective is to roll into the crook of your assailant's elbow and onto your stomach to break the hold. Maneuver your body away to the opposite side of his choking elbow to create some space to turn back into the crook of his elbow, create separation, and defeat the choke. Note: the turn onto your stomach must be forceful. The goal is to turn and end up facing the assailant, allowing counterattacks such as eye gouges, knees, and other combatives. "About-facing" your torso will break his grip. *Do not in any way use your hands to push his legs away, as this leaves your neck and throat exposed.*

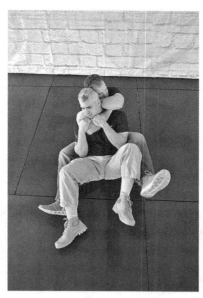

To ward off the assailant's hooks, raise your right leg to prevent him from sinking his leg hooks into you while keeping your elbows at your sides to further prevent him from sinking his hooks in.

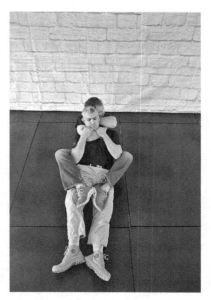

Keep your chin tucked, and with both of your arms yank down on his choking arm prior to his sinking the choke. If he sinks the choke with his right arm, you must yank down on his right arm just below the elbow and just above the elbow at the "V" of his arm. A second option is to yank down on his right arm just above his wrist with your right hand and use your left hand to remove his left hand from the back of your head. Use your torso and legs to push back by bridging to place your entire body weight on him. Once you have shifted your weight back, if he has sunk his hooks, you must flatten your legs out and bring them together while still using your core upper-body strength to resist the choke. You must force the assailant on his back with your torso weight firmly against him so he cannot lean back and apply additional choking pressure.

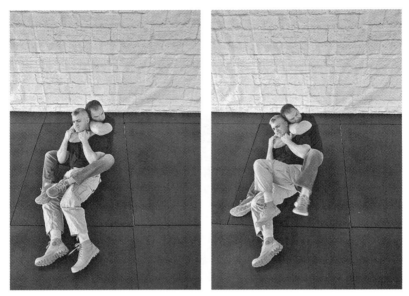

As you resist the choke, slide your left leg up and through to grapevine around one of his hooks. Then slide your right leg over the other hook.

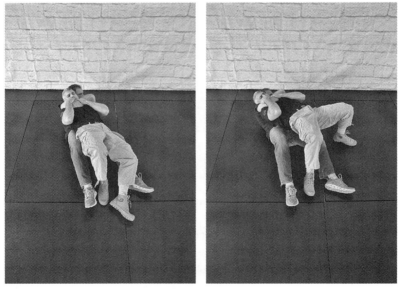

Once you have slid your hips out, still pinning him with your torso, bridge again by raising your body on the balls of your feet. Slide your hips perpendicular to the opponent's torso and begin breaking the choke hold. Counterattack the groin to create further separation and continue to pin him to the ground as you begin your defensive torso turn.

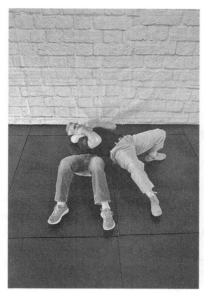 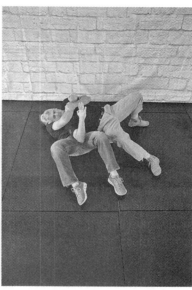

Use your body weight, enhanced by the bridge, to maneuver your body away approximately 90 degrees (to the opposite side of his choking elbow) to create space. Once you have broken the initial choke, deliver strong elbow strikes to his groin.

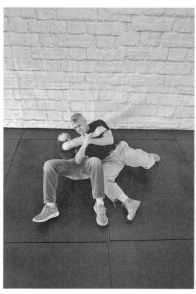 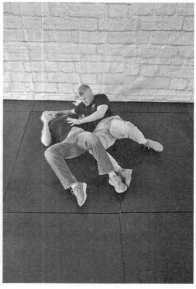

Once you have created separation and released his initial grip, turn forcefully onto your stomach to end up facing the assailant, which will allow counterattacks such as eye gouges, knees, and other combatives. In about-facing your torso, you will break his entire grip while continuing to counterattack.

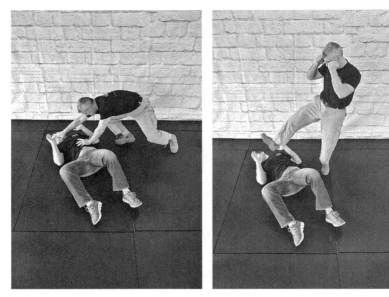

Get up by continuing to place pressure on his head and body, and finish with kicks and stomps as necessary.

Note: if your assailant is able to sink his leg hooks, a third option is to keep your chin tucked and use both arms to remove his left hand from the back of your head to counterattack with a straight armbar over your shoulder. Be sure you have defended against the choke adequately before going on the counteroffensive. Sliding your hips out will increase pressure on the arm. Be sure to keep his thumb pointed up. Note: you must execute this move quickly because both of your hands are committed, leaving you vulnerable.

Rear Mounted Naked Choke Defense against a Figure-Four Leg Lock

This type of choke—like all chokes—is extremely dangerous. Of course, the best way to defend it—again, as with all chokes—is not to get put into it. As with the preceding rear naked choke defense, do not let the assailant get his legs around you, especially when he is attempting a figure-four type of lock. A strong opponent with long legs can use a figure-four hold to hamper your mobility, break your ribs, and literally squeeze the life out of you, using both his upper body and lower body.

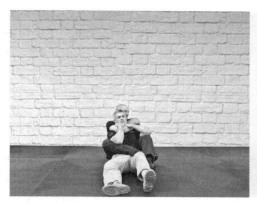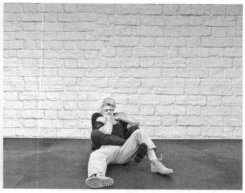

To defend this type of choke, use the same defensive options as covered previously in tucking your chin and exerting counterpressure at the "V" of his elbow, except you must wrap your nearside leg around the assailant's dangling lower leg to apply a vicious ankle lock.

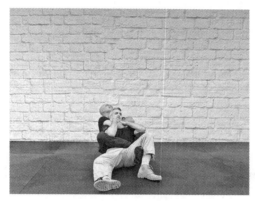

Once your nearside leg is hooked over, extend your leg to exert breaking pressure on his ankle joint. Be sure to maintain steady counterpressure against his choke until he either releases the figure four or the choke. Defeat the choke as covered in the previous defense, Rear Naked Choke Defense (Warding Off the Hooks).

Defense against the Rear Mounted Naked Choke When Facedown

This is an extremely dangerous position to find yourself in and should be preempted or prevented if possible. There are professional assailants who, once they have this position, will not let go. So, the key is to avoid and prevent being placed in this dangerous choke. But if you find yourself facedown with an assailant on your back attempting to apply a rear naked choke variation, you must immediately tuck your chin and apply counterpressure. Because of the position, you may have to secure the assailant at the wrist and upper forearm next to the elbow hinge to apply counterpressure. The goal once again is to turn and end up facing the assailant, allowing counterattacks such as eye gouges, knees, and other combatives. "About-facing" your torso will break his grip. Once you create enough separation to breathe comfortably, counterattack his eyes and groin, followed by retzev.

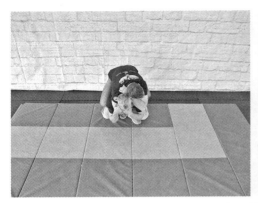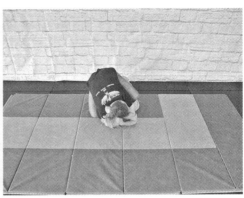

To release, maintain counterpressure against his choking arm. As you resist the choke, try to rise to your knees.

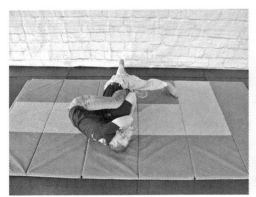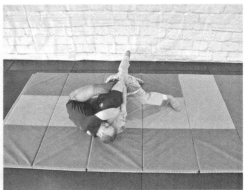

If you can rise to your knees, as you begin to buck the assailant forward, scissor your legs outward in the direction of the choking arm. In other words, if the assailant is applying the choke with his right arm across or around your neck, you will scissor your legs out and to your right. Similar to the rear-mounted choke with your back to the ground, this scissoring action allows you the best possibility of breaking his grip. Continue to turn into the assailant.

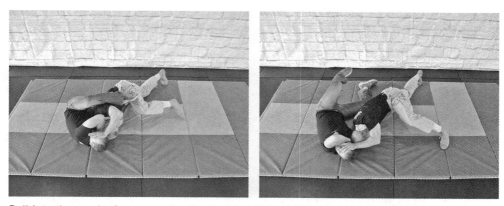

Roll into the crook of your assailant's elbow and forcefully onto your stomach to break the hold while attacking his eyes. Maneuver your body away to the opposite side of his choking elbow to create space.

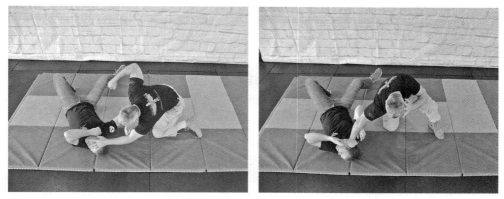

Continue to turn into the crook of his elbow to create separation and defeat the choke.

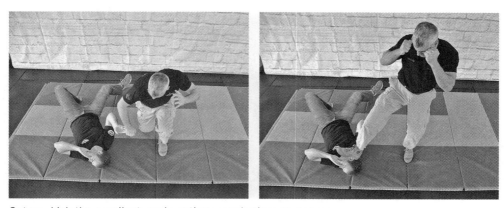

Get up, kick the assailant, and continue combatives as necessary.

Defending the Guard

If you maintain proper upright body position, the opponent's groin is open to strikes.

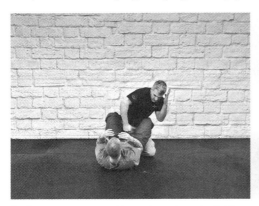 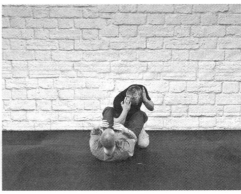

Strike your opponent's groin using straight punches (depicted), vertical elbows (depicted), or hammer fists. You may also trap one or both of the opponent's arms while delivering simultaneous combatives.

Defending the Guard if the Opponent Pulls the Defender In

If your opponent successfully breaks your posture and clinches your head, use thumb gouges to the eyes to disengage, followed by retzev.

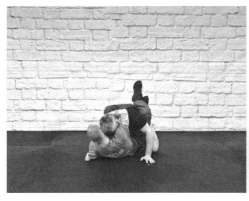 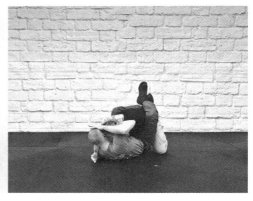

Immediately insert one or both of your thumbs into the opponent's eye sockets.

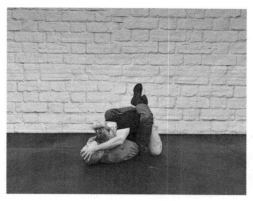

Extend both of your arms and use the rule of thumb that if you find the cheekbone, you find the eyeball. Press your thumbs into the assailant's eyeballs to break the attack. Continue to counter-attack anatomical vulnerabilities as opportune.

Neck Crank from the High Guard

The neck crank from the guard can have serious consequences for your adversary, especially if you keep your legs pincered. (Note: this powerful technique is also readily available from the inside clinch.) While on your back, you have drawn your adversary into you, facing you between your pincered legs.

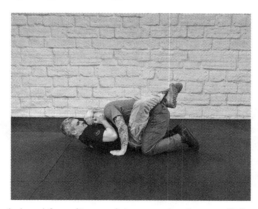

Securing your adversary's head from its rear into your chest, you will force your adversary's chin sideways while your other arm reaches around to secure his forehead or nearside eye socket. Clamp down on his torso with your closed guard and torque or crank his neck forcefully to the side.

Krav maga recognizes that you may end up on your back in a fight. So you must be capable of defending against all manner of combatives, especially strikes and chokes. When you close your guard by wrapping one ankle around the other, and if you react quickly to protect your groin by pulling your adversary's torso close to you, the guard position offers the opportunity to deploy a weapon secured on your leg.

You must maneuver quickly because your groin is exposed to counterattack. By immediately forcing the assailant's head into your torso while burying your head against your shoulder or biceps to protect your eyes, deploy your weapon.

Offenses from the Rear Mount

When there is no choice but to go to the ground, "taking" the adversary's back—placing your chest to his back with his torso between your legs—is the most advantageous position, provided you are not facing multiple opponents. This is because you have an array of combative strikes and chokes at your disposal, including elbows and forearm strikes to the back of the neck, eye gouges, and heel kicks to your adversary's groin and abdomen. Keep in mind that if an adversary takes your back, all of these offensive tactics may be used against you.

Rear Naked Choke with Heel Kicks

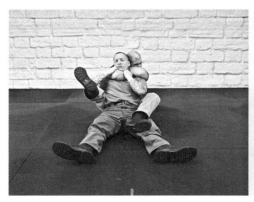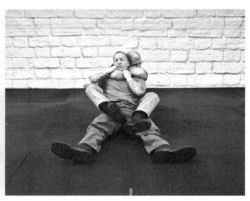

As you apply the choke and sink your hooks, use your heels to deliver withering, debilitating strikes to his groin.

Rear Naked Choke with Eye Rake

If the adversary is resisting your choke, rake his eyes with your non-choking arm to expose his throat and neck to apply the choke.

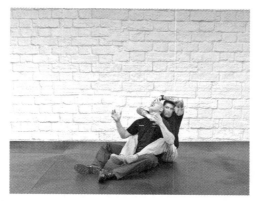

To facilitate exposing the opponent's neck to apply a choke, you may embed your fingers in the opponent's eyes and rake his head back. Significant pressure applied to the eye sockets when pulling to the rear will force the opponent to pick his head up, thereby lifting his chin in an attempt to alleviate the pressure.

Rear Naked Choke with Philtrum Rake (Not Depicted)

To facilitate exposing the opponent's neck to apply a choke, you may use your fore-finger to lift underneath the opponent's nose (his philtrum) to force his head back. Signif-icant pressure applied underneath the philtrum when pulling rearward will force the opponent to pick his head up, thereby lifting his chin in an attempt to alleviate the pres-sure. Note: you must apply this technique quickly and precisely to avoid being bitten.

Boxing the Ears and Striking with Elbows

Highly effective combatives involving the ear also include "boxing" the ears with palm heel strikes or using elbow strikes to the base of the skull or back of the head.

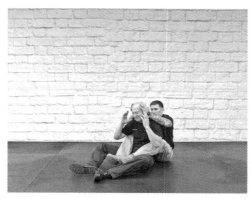

Palm heel strikes to the ears.

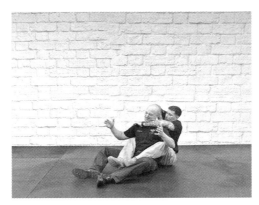

Elbow strikes to the back of the head.

Counters to Defensive Measures against Your Rear Naked Choke Attempt

If the adversary defends your rear naked choke attempt by yanking down on your choking arm, you may use your other arm to apply the choke. Note: you may also grab your own clothing, reinforcing the hold, while repositioning your other arm underneath his chin to execute an opposite arm choke. Basically, you are switching one choking arm for the other.

Offenses from the Mount

When obtaining the mount, do not sit on your adversary. Keep your weight settled high on his chest to maintain balance and control his arms. Protect your groin with a forward lean. Your knees must provide good balance platforms as you hook your heels into the side of your adversary. In addition, your knees should be close to his torso and as high as possible toward his armpits to limit his striking and evasive abilities. (In defending the mount, as a countertechnique, keep your elbows in to prevent the adversary from riding up the torso.)

Mount with Forearm Groin Shield

Place yourself in the best possible position to strike and control while defending your groin by grabbing onto the assailant's shirt right in front of your groin.

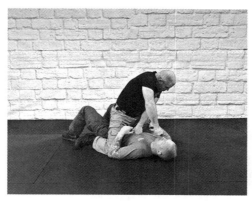

Place your forearm in front of your groin to provide a partial shield, allowing you to attack with your free arm. This may be achieved by securing the assailant by the shirt with your weak-side arm to form a partial defensive shield against strikes to your groin. With your strong-side arm, pummel him with punches, palm heel strikes, vertical elbow drops, and forearm shivers.

Another strong option is to control the adversary's arms, which provides two tactical advantages: you can rain combative strikes down on his head and throat with impunity along with armbar options and chokes, and you can prevent him from striking your groin. Even if you do not control your adversary's arms, you can still pierce his defenses to attack his head and throat. From the mount you have more mobility, and gravity is on your side as you deliver withering combatives. It is highly advantageous to keep your adversary's back pinned to the ground to limit his escape options.

You can also position yourself with one knee on an adversary's arm while trapping his other arm to facilitate combatives. This option also allows for armbar variations against the adversary's free arm. For example, you can transition from a control hold to an armbar combined with a throat grab. For the armbar throat-grab technique on the ground, you will trap one of the adversary's arms with your knee or reverse the mount across into a far-side armbar.

The following points will help you to maintain and use the mount long enough to deploy a cold or hot weapon:

- To maintain the mount, you must develop good balance to counter the adversary's body turns and push releases and to deploy your cold and hot weapons. One of the most common defenses is for the adversary to buck or throw you using his hips to bridge. Note: this is a krav maga defense against a substandard mount.
- If your adversary wishes to roll on his stomach, let him. Loosen your legs slightly to allow the adversary's movement while deploying your weapon; if you tighten them he can throw you or roll you over.

- If your adversary tries to close the distance between you by using a "bear hug" from the bottom, you can use eye gouges (similar to the standing defense) or apply a painful arm brace to the jaw and throat by bracing his face across the jaw with your forearm or using the palm heel of one or both of your arms. The same technique will work if your opponent tries to grab your neck. Insert your arm as a brace against his throat and jaw.

Trapping the Adversary's Arms for Weapon Deployment

Trapping an adversary's arm or arms takes away both his ability to defend and to counterattack you, specifically your groin. You can deliver extreme punishment from this advantageous position and readily deploy your weapon. Trap your adversary's arm by securing it firmly against your body with the inside of your forearm (both arms can be trapped in this way as well).

CHAPTER 4

Impact-Weapon Combatives and Defenses

Impact-weapon attacks can come from a myriad of angles and directions. For an unarmed defender, the three fundamental options in defending against an impact-weapon attack are as follows:

1. Close the distance between you and the assailant while deflecting-redirecting the attack.
2. Disengage until you recognize the correct timing for closing the distance.
3. Retreat straightaway.

For any object thrown at you, you need to use a body defense to make it miss. As covered in the second part of this chapter, if you are armed with an impact weapon yourself, close the distance between you and the assailant while deflecting-redirecting the attack and then seamlessly and immediately moving to a counterattack. For impact weapons, we will focus on four common types of impact-weapon attacks: overhead, overhead off-angle, side-swing, and lower-quadrant attacks.

For security-conscious civilians who are not legally permitted to carry a firearm, or for those who are but may choose a lesser force option for a particular scenario, an elongated flashlight is a superb impact weapon. I prefer the MagLite® six C-cell model and carry it with me in my vehicle. The flashlight is also, of course, useful as a flashlight. This is the model depicted in a number of the photos.

Impact Weapon against Upper- and Lower-Body Strikes

Impact Weapon against a Straight Punch

Impact weapons may be used with great effect against upper-body and lower-body attacks. If you have an extended impact weapon and an assailant is foolhardy enough to attempt a straight punch against you, use the impact weapon combined with a body defense. Sidestep his incoming punch, moving to the deadside, while intercepting the punching arm, attacking the green-zone targets of his incoming arm and forward leg, as this law enforcement example demonstrates.

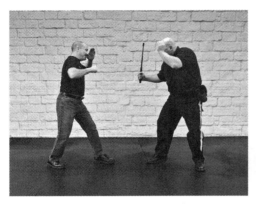 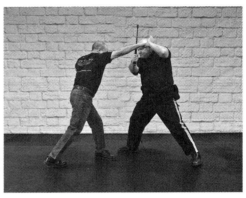

From a ready position, with your right leg and arm forward, move off the line of attack by side-stepping diagonally forward, away from his incoming strike, while simultaneously striking his incoming arm. Keep your other hand and arm defensively positioned in a gunt, an angled elbow block defense (see *Krav Maga Weapon Defenses* [YMAA, 2012], pages 110–111). This will allow you to respond if the assailant tries to attack you with his other arm.

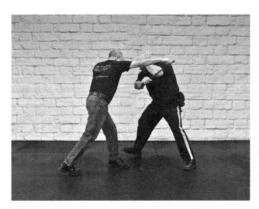 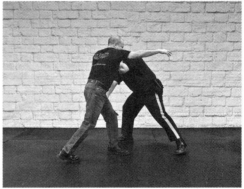

After battering the assailant's punching arm, redirect the weapon using a backhand strike to the assailant's nearside leg.

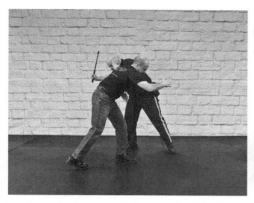 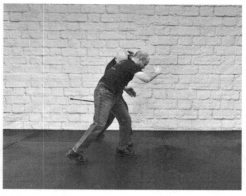

Continue to move past the assailant to his deadside to allow additional green-zone strikes as necessary.

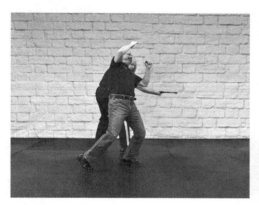 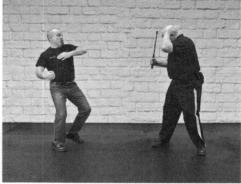

Also as necessary, deliver a strike to the back of the legs (provided it is justified within a use-of-force protocol).

Another alternative is for the defender to simply use timing and the impact weapon's length to make a direct thrust at the assailant's vulnerable anatomy.

Impact Weapon against a Hook Punch

This defense is nearly the same as defending against a straight punch when in an opposite outlet stance. Note: this is an integral part of krav maga—one technique or solution to thwart a number of similar attacks. Once again, if you have an extended impact weapon and an assailant is foolhardy enough to attempt a straight punch against you, use the impact weapon combined with a body defense. Sidestep his incoming punch, moving to his deadside, while intercepting the punching arm and attacking the green-zone targets of his incoming arm. If necessary, you may attack his forward leg too.

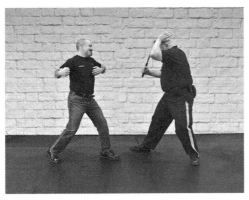 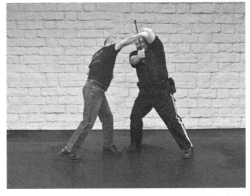

From a ready position, with your right leg and arm forward, move off the line of attack by side-stepping diagonally forward, away from his incoming strike, while simultaneously and forcefully striking his incoming arm.

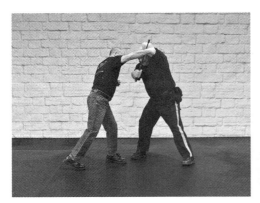 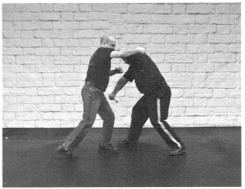

After battering the assailant's punching arm, redirect the weapon using a natural backhand strike to the assailant's nearside leg. Keep your other hand and arm defensively positioned in a gunt, should the assailant try to attack you with his other arm.

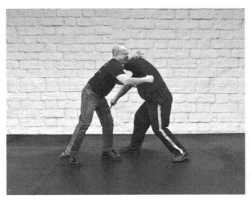 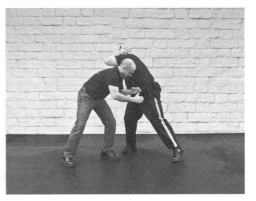

Continue to move past the assailant to his deadside to allow additional green-zone strikes as necessary.

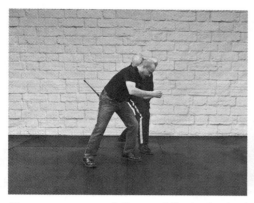 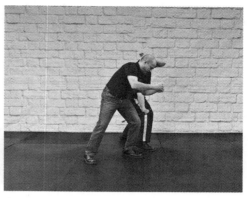

Also as necessary, deliver a strike to the back of the legs (provided it is justified within your use-of-force protocol).

Impact Weapon against a Straight Kick

If you have an extended impact weapon and an assailant is imprudent enough to attempt a kick against you, use the impact weapon combined with a body defense. Side-step his incoming straight kick by moving to the deadside. As you step off the line of attack, intercept and batter the kicking leg, followed by additional green-zone targets as necessary.

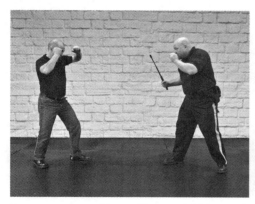 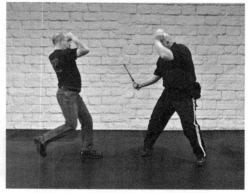

From a ready position, with your right leg and arm forward, move off the line of attack by side-stepping diagonally forward, away from his incoming kick, while preparing to strike the outstretched leg.

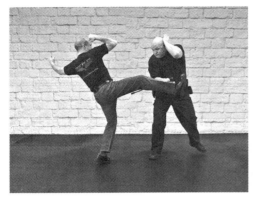 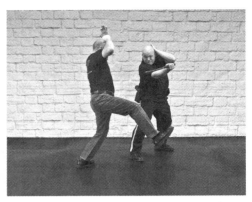

After battering the assailant's leg, redirect the weapon to administer a natural backhand strike to the assailant's thigh.

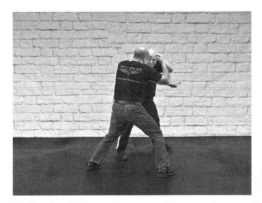 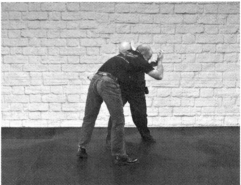

Strike the thigh and keep moving past the assailant to reassess or to assert control. Move to the assailant's deadside to allow additional green-zone strikes as necessary.

Note: an alternative defense is to use an inverted impact-weapon swing, which moves you advantageously to the assailant's deadside. This defense is depicted next.

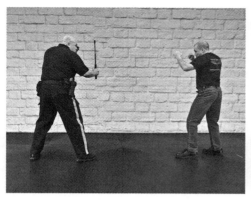 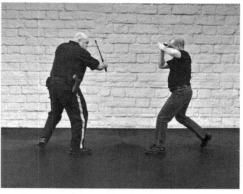

From a ready position, with your right leg and arm forward, move off the line of attack by stepping forward with the left leg while simultaneously striking the outstretched leg using an inverted strike.

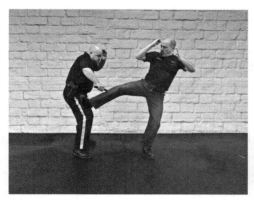 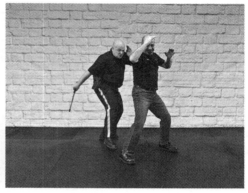

After battering the assailant's leg, redirect the weapon using a backhand strike to the assailant's thigh and continue to move past the assailant.

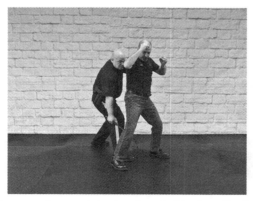

You may use the impact weapon to assert dominant control by thrusting it between the assailant's legs.

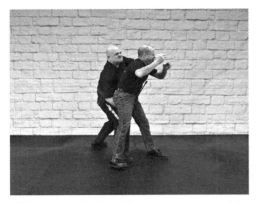 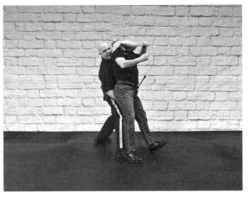

Lift up with the impact weapon while applying a face bar, taking care to force his head to the side. Be careful not to place your hand or arm across the assailant's mouth, as he may attempt to bite you. Note: this form of restraint is aggressive and may be outside a particular use-of-force protocol.

Impact Weapon against a Tackle or Two-Leg Takedown

If you have an impact weapon and an assailant is foolish enough to attempt a tackle against you, simply use the impact weapon's length to direct a thrust against the assailant's vulnerable anatomy. If you are armed with a long gun, you may use it as an impact weapon, combined with a body defense. Sidestep your adversary's attempted tackle while moving to the deadside, at the same time intercepting and jamming the opponent's lowered head, neck, and trapezius as he drops for the tackle. (See Long-Gun Thrust with Sidestep against a Tackle in chapter 5 and Twelve O'Clock Modified Sprawl in chapter 9.) After jamming and thwarting the assailant's progress, use the impact weapon as necessary to neutralize the threat.

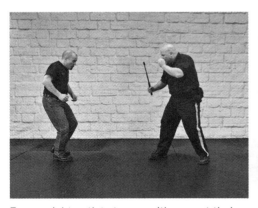 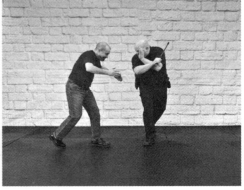

From a right outlet stance, with correct timing, move off the line of attack by taking a step back with the rear left leg while simultaneously striking the nearside leg.

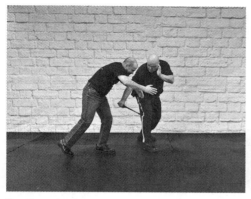 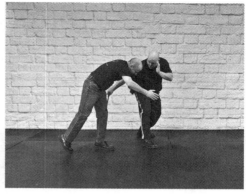

Continue to move past the assailant as you strike his leg.

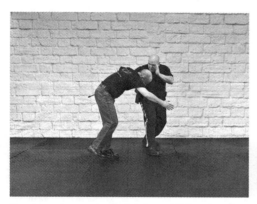 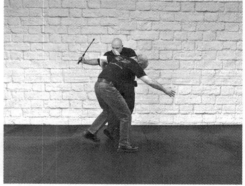

Keep moving and administer additional strikes as necessary.

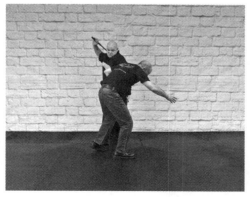

If necessary (and justified), continue to strike green-zone targets.

Head Strike Variation (Deadly Force Encounter)

An alternative defense, which you can use if you believe yourself to be in a *deadly force encounter*, including facing multiple assailants, is to sidestep and strike to the head, or "red zone," instead of the thigh. You can also strike him on the upper back if your sidestep is effective and reach allows.

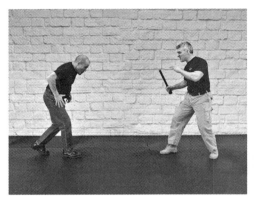 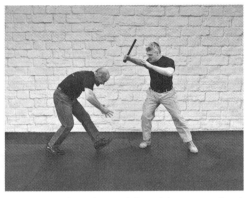

From a right outlet stance, with correct timing, move off the line of attack by taking a step back with the rear left leg while simultaneously striking to the head.

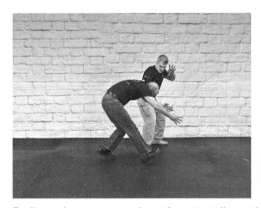 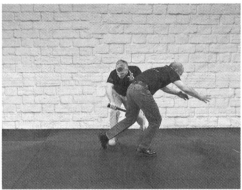

Redirect the weapon and continue to strike to the knee to hobble the assailant.

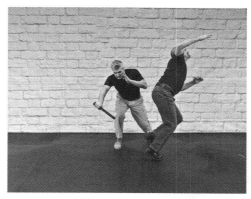

Continue to move past the assailant out of the danger zone and prepare to confront additional threats.

A third defense is to simply thrust the impact weapon into the incoming assailant's face.

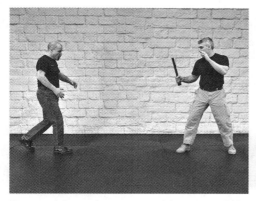 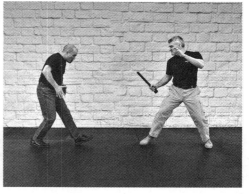

From a right outlet stance, with correct timing, thrust the impact weapon into the assailant's face as he closes on you.

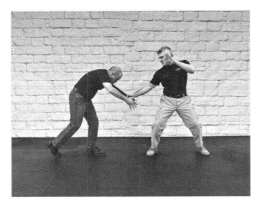

To maximize the strike, pivot slightly on your forward leg to engage the hips and upper body in concert.

Short Impact Weapon against Short Impact Weapon

Krav maga's defenses using an impact weapon against an impact-weapon threat or assault (impact vs. impact) follow many of the same tenets that apply when defending open handed, or unarmed. The key, whenever possible, is to use a deflection-redirection combined with a body defense while stepping off the line of attack. As you step off the line, use counterstrikes that naturally follow from a deflection of the opponent's impact weapon—preferably to the assailant's head, eyes, face, neck, and throat. You may also use impact-weapon strikes in combination with kicks for retzev, using your legs, free arm, and impact weapon. The focus here is on using a "short" impact weapon such as a flashlight or baton, although an improvised weapon like a rolled-up magazine or umbrella would work as well. Many of these impact-weapon vs. impact-weapon defenses are simply modified when using an impact weapon to defend against an edged weapon, as you will see.

Note: the following tactics assume the defender does not have access to a firearm.

Impact Weapon against Overhead Impact Weapon

The assailant has the impact weapon in his right hand and is facing you. This attack can involve tremendous force as the assailant presses all of his weight into the attack while using gravity to his advantage. The IKMA curriculum has two defensive options against an overhead type of attack. These options would work against a straight punch or hook punch; however, the follow-through or follow-up must take use of force into consideration. A punch, while it could theoretically do severe damage or kill you (especially if delivered by a trained fighter), generally does not present the same danger to you as an impact weapon or edged weapon.

For either defensive option, stand with the impact weapon in your strong-side hand with the same-side leg forward. In other words, a right-handed defender will stand in a forward outlet stance. Either defense requires the defender to step off line and attack the assailant's incoming arm, continuing with retzev counterattacks to neutralize the threat. By design, you will notice a similarity when comparing impact-weapon vs. impact-weapon defenses to impact-weapon vs. edged-weapon defenses. You will also once again see krav maga's emphasis on a few core tactics to defend against a multitude of threats and attacks.

Deflect-redirect the assailant's overhead impact-weapon attack using a variation of the 360-degree parry while angling your impact weapon slightly down and away to make the opponent's impact weapon glance off and away. This provides a twofold tactical advantage:

1. It allows you to lessen the impact on your defending arm.
2. It frees your impact weapon for an immediate counterattack using a backswing strike (following a natural strike progression) to the assailant's head or neck with the impact weapon.

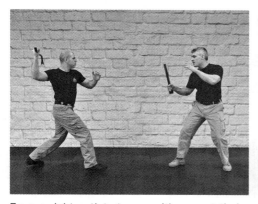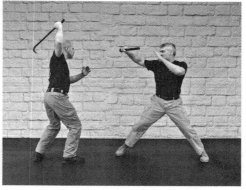

From a right outlet stance, with correct timing, move off the line of attack by stepping diagonally and forward slightly. This movement blades the body and begins to angle your impact weapon above your head, with the tip pointed down to deflect his incoming strike.

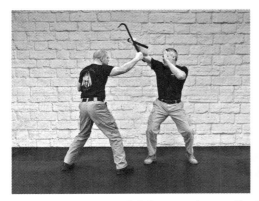
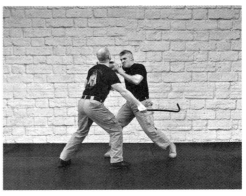

Angling your weapon slightly, meet the assailant's weapon and let it slide off your weapon. Your impact weapon is both tactically and strategically positioned to continue with a horizontal strike to the assailant's head. Continue with your forward movement to make the strike.

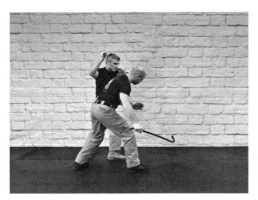
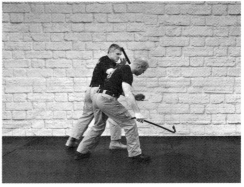

Using tai-sabaki footwork, continue to move past the assailant. This footwork allows you to deliver another strong strike to the assailant's head with additional combatives, including a kick to the groin or side kick to the knee, followed by additional impact strikes if the assailant continues to present a threat.

Impact Weapon against Overhead Impact Weapon, Variation

This alternative defense may be used when

1. you are close to the assailant;
2. you cannot sidestep (such as when you are in close confines or standing against a wall);

3. you are in a multiple-adversary situation and you must keep the defender to the deadside and away from other adversaries; and

4. the assailant comes from an oblique angle (off-angle attack).

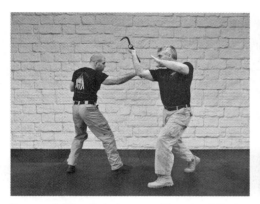 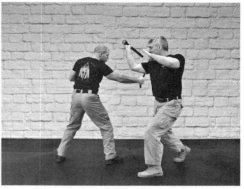

From a right outlet stance, with correct timing, move off the line of attack by stepping forward with your rear left leg. This blades your body while simultaneously angling your impact weapon above your head with the tip pointed down, keeping your other hand up as well. Strengthen your arm and grip to meet the assailant's incoming weapon. Let the attacking weapon glance off your weapon.

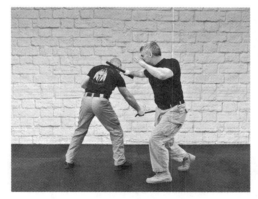

Immediately rotate your weapon approximately 180 degrees, using the torque of the rotation to counterattack the assailant's head. Your impact weapon is positioned to continue with a rotating horizontal strike to the assailant's head. Rotate your hips clockwise while pivoting on the balls of your feet to maximize the impact. You may continue the counterattack with a side kick to the assailant's nearside knee. Continue to administer combatives with the impact weapon until the adversary is no longer a threat.

Note: the current IKMA curriculum does not advocate gripping a short impact weapon with two hands to stop an overhead attack. While this is possible to defend the attack, it is always preferable to also step off the line of attack for a double measure of safety. In any event, for this technique, whether remaining stationary to absorb the full impact of his incoming strike or stepping off the line with two hands on your impact weapon, be sure to deliver a simultaneous or near-simultaneous kick in keeping with krav maga's principles of combined defense and attack.

Impact Weapon Straight Thrust against Overhead Impact Weapon

With exceptional timing, a third alternative defense may be used to sidestep the overhead attack and thrust your impact weapon into the assailant's head.

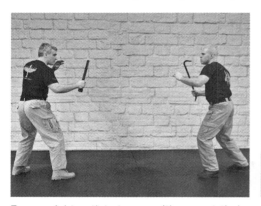 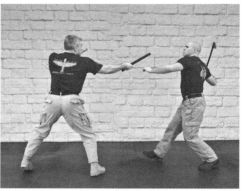

From a right outlet stance, with correct timing, move off the line of attack by stepping diagonally and forward slightly off the line of attack. Your rear left leg steps back slightly while you simultaneously angle your impact weapon to thrust it into the assailant's neck or head, keeping your other hand up as well.

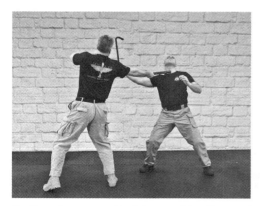 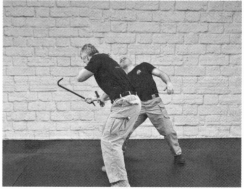

Continue to counterattack by smashing the assailant's weapon arm to force him to drop his weapon.

Impact Weapon against Impact Weapon Forehand Side-Swing Attack

This defense, once again by design, is similar to defending against a hook punch, edged-weapon slash, or hook stab. This defense is also notably similar to previous impact-weapon straight stab defenses in footwork and weapon deployment. On interception, your impact weapon is positioned following a natural strike progression to continue with a horizontal strike to the assailant's head.

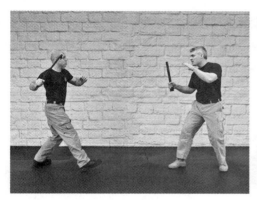 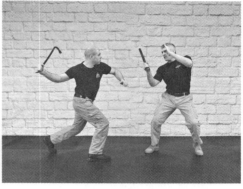

From a right outlet stance, with correct timing, move off the line of attack by stepping diagonally and forward slightly as you step your rear (left) leg back slightly and simultaneously angle your impact weapon to intercept his incoming side swing, keeping your other hand up as well.

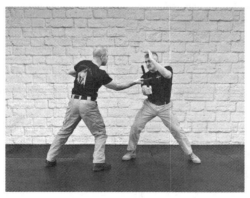

Strengthen your arm and grip to meet the assailant's incoming weapon.

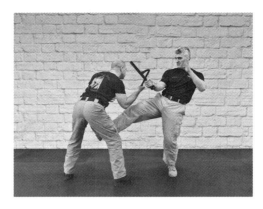

As you intercept the side swing, you may use a small shuffle front kick. Step forward slightly with your rear leg and use your front let to launch the kick into the assailant's groin.

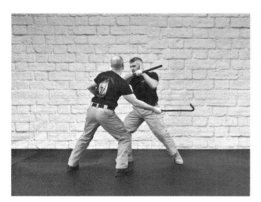 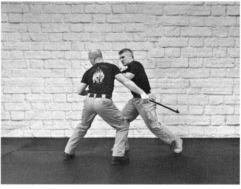

On intercepting the strike, immediately continue to move your impact weapon along a horizontal plane to strike the assailant in the head. Rotate your hips clockwise while pivoting on the balls of your feet to maximize the strike.

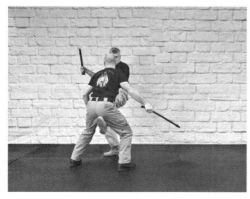 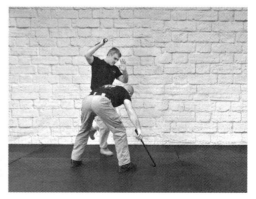

You may continue the counterattack with a straight kick to the assailant's groin using your rear (more proximate) leg. Continue to move past the assailant using a tai-sabaki step. This step moves you away from the assailant while still keeping him in front of you.

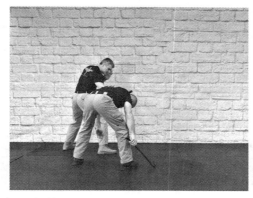

Continue with additional combatives as necessary.

Impact Weapon against Impact Weapon High Backhand Side Swing

The goal is to burst inside the arc of the impact weapon's back slash and jam or smash the assailant's weapon arm with your impact weapon. To close on the assailant, switch your stance, keeping your weapon perpendicular to the ground. At the same time, your free arm is parallel to your weapon to help jam the assailant at the shoulder as he commences the swing. Parry and trap the assailant's arm while executing impact-weapon combatives to his head and weapon arm.

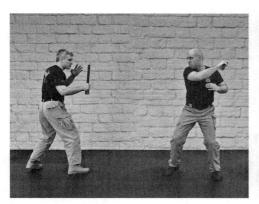
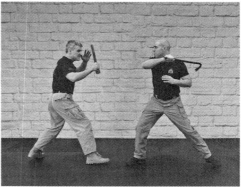

From a right outlet stance and with correct timing, step forward with both legs, maintaining the same distance between your feet, to intercept his incoming strike. Keep your impact weapon vertical, holding it tightly and strengthening your arm.

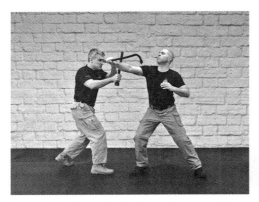 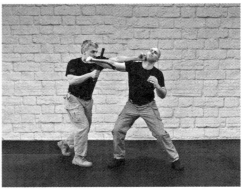

Intercept and smash his incoming arm with your impact weapon. As simultaneously as possible, deliver an inverted punch to the assailant's head.

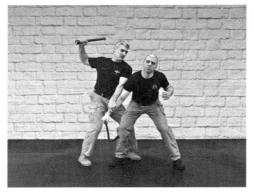

Next use your free hand to clamp down on the assailant's weapon arm, placing your body weight on it to further immobilize it. Continue with additional combatives as necessary.

Impact Weapon against Impact Weapon High Backhand Side Swing, Variation

As you recognize the assailant's impending backswing, burst into the assailant with your impact weapon parallel to the ground and the tip aimed at the assailant's neck or head. In essence, this defense is preempting the assailant's ability to deliver a strike by striking him first. Timing, as always, is crucial.

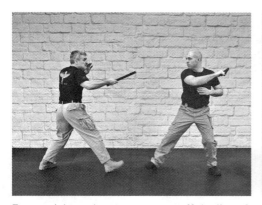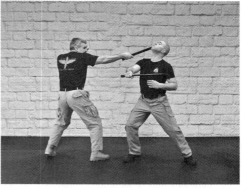

From a right outlet stance, move off the line of attack by stepping diagonally and slightly forward to blade your body and angle your impact weapon to thrust it into the assailant's neck or head, keeping your other hand up as well.

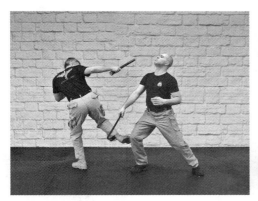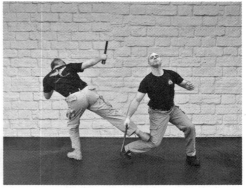

Continue to counterattack. One option is to destroy the assailant's knee with a low side kick. Of course, you continue to administer strikes with your impact weapon.

Impact-Weapon Defense When Handgun Is Inoperable

If you are facing an impact-weapon threat but your handgun is either inoperable or out of ammunition, you may revert to krav maga's open-handed defense and use your handgun as an impact weapon. Close the distance to intercept and deflect-redirect the impact weapon harmlessly over your shoulder while thrusting the handgun muzzle into the assailant's throat, jaw, or face. At the same time, you trap the weapon arm to remove the weapon from the assailant's grip while delivering more retzev combatives.

Essentially, you are diving or bursting into your assailant with the same-side arm and leg to close the distance while deflecting-redirecting the strike and simultaneously counter-striking. Another way to think about aligning your deflecting-redirecting arm is to stand in a neutral stance and extend your arm directly to meet an imaginary incoming attack. The deflecting-stabbing defense, when timed correctly and with proper interception alignment, will redirect the object harmlessly along your arm over your head, glancing off your back. Time the defense and counterpunch together.

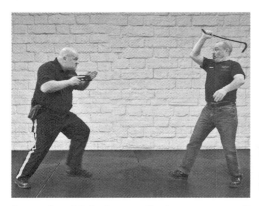
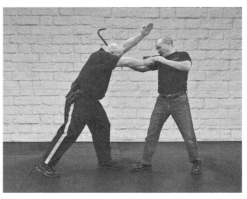

As you burst into the assailant, proper arm alignment requires a slight curve in your hand that will intercept the attack. Keep the fingers together and the thumb firmly against your hand; if you leave the thumb out, it might get broken by the weapon.

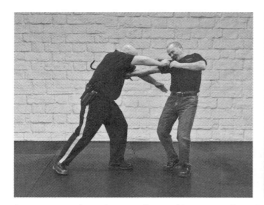
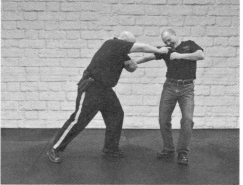

As you move into the assailant with your redirection and simultaneous cold-weapon strike, without breaking contact with the assailant's arm, loop your deflecting-stabbing arm over the assailant's impact-weapon arm to secure the impact-weapon arm. You may continue your counterattack with a foreleg kick, multiple knee strikes to the groin, or use your handgun again as a cold weapon. The most popular method to remove the impact weapon is to use a 180-degree step (tai-sabaki) with your right foot to break or rip the impact weapon away from his hand without taking your eyes off him.

Off-Angle Overhead Impact Defense When Handgun Is Inoperable

If an assailant attempts an off-angle swing toward your right side, a variation of the out-of-battery defense is to deflect his incoming weapon with your gun hand.

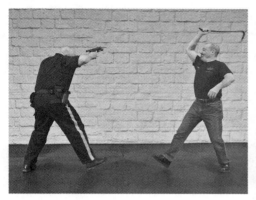 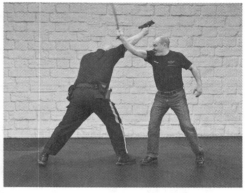

As you burst into the assailant, proper arm alignment requires a slight curve in the hand that will intercept the attack. Point the firearm slightly away to position your hand correctly to "spear" his incoming arm.

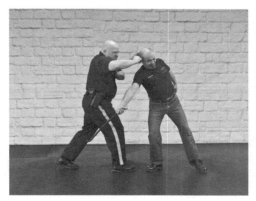

As soon as the impact weapon glides over your shoulder, strike the assailant in the head with your weapon.

Impact Weapon Two-Handed Side-Swing Defense When Handgun Is Inoperable

The defense against a side-swing attack is similar to the first overhead-attack defense we examined. Again, the emphasis is on one defense that will defeat a myriad of attacks. If, for example, the assailant were to feint an overhead attack and then quickly change the angle of the weapon to make it a side swing, the defense works either way.

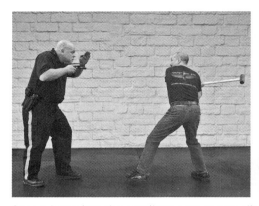 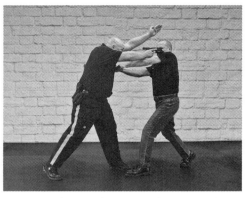

As you burst into the assailant, proper arm alignment requires a slight curve in the hand that will intercept the overhead attack. By closing on the assailant, you will absorb the strike on your left lateral muscle. Strike the assailant in the face with your inoperable handgun in a cold-weapon capacity.

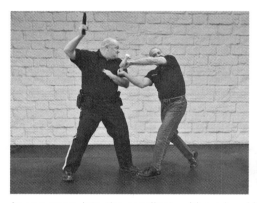 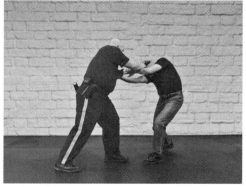

As you move into the assailant, without breaking contact with the assailant's arm, loop your deflecting-stabbing arm over the assailant's impact-weapon arm to secure the impact-weapon arm. Continue your counterattack with additional handgun strikes as necessary. The most popular method to remove the impact weapon is to use a 180-degree step (tai-sabaki) with your right foot to break or rip the impact weapon away from his hand without taking your eyes off him.

Impact Weapon Two-Handed Side-Swing Defense When Handgun Is Inoperable, Variation

A third option is to close the distance against a side swing (or overhead attack) with your arms in a wedge formation. This modification exemplifies krav maga's key tenet of combined simultaneous defense and attack.

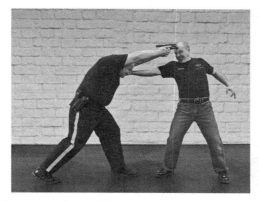

Using a two-handed grip on your inoperable handgun, your arms are naturally positioned in a wedged to intercept and counterattack at the same time. Once again, proper arm alignment requires a slight curve in the hand that will intercept the overhead attack. By closing on the assailant, you will absorb the strike on your lateral muscle.

Impact Weapon against Edged-Weapon Attack

Krav maga's defenses when using an impact weapon against an edged-weapon threat or assault (impact edged), as noted and by design, follow most of the same principles involved in defending open handed or the previous impact-weapon impact-weapon defenses. Again, the goal is to learn a few proven tactics and adapt them to any given situation. Try whenever possible to use a deflection-redirection combined with a body defense, stepping off the line of attack. In addition, you deliver simultaneous counterstrikes, preferably to the assailant's head, eyes, face, neck, or throat.

The focus here is using a designated impact weapon, although an improvised weapon such as a rolled-up magazine or umbrella would work as well. If your defense is imperfect and you are stabbed or wounded, it is imperative that you press your defense and counterattack. Note that krav maga defenses against an edged weapon, broken bottle, or syringe are essentially the same.

The following techniques focus on defenses against the most common types of edged-weapon attacks. To be sure, not every angle or direction is covered. Absorb the principles and apply them against other variations. Use good common sense along with a little trial and error in your training.

Impact Defenses against an Assailant Posturing with an Edged Weapon (Midlevel)

The IKMA curriculum has two defensive preemptive options against an assailant posturing with a knife held at midlevel. For both variations, the assailant faces you with the edged weapon in his right hand.

Windmill Variation

For the first variation, you may use an "outside" continuous windmill defense to break his arm, "defanging the snake," or hit him in the head. The key is to keep the impact weapon moving continuously and offensively.

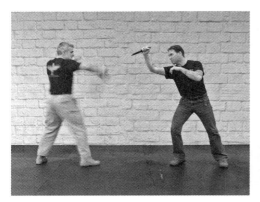 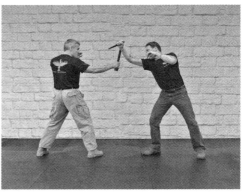

Keep the impact weapon rotating clockwise in a continuous fast rotation. Close enough distance on the assailant to use the impact weapon's reach.

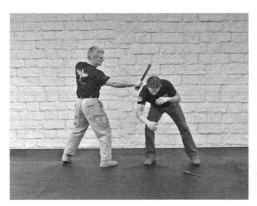 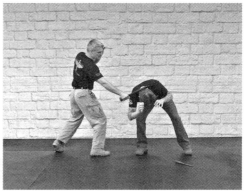

Continue the rotation to administer additional combatives as necessary to end the threat.

Straight Stab Sidestep and Attack

For the variation, target the weapon arm and then continue your attack as necessary. On interception, your impact weapon is positioned to follow a natural strike progression ending in a horizontal strike to the assailant's head.

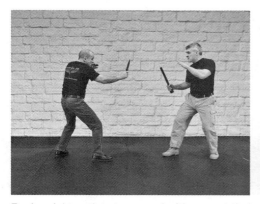 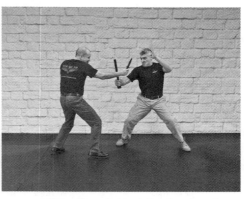

From a right outlet stance and with correct timing, move off the line of attack by stepping diagonally and forward slightly to blade your body and angle your weapon, and smash the assailant's knife arm. (Note the similarity by design to Impact Weapon against Impact Weapon Forehand Side-Swing Attack.)

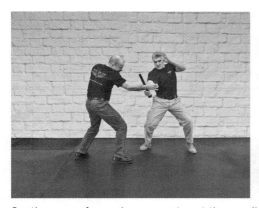 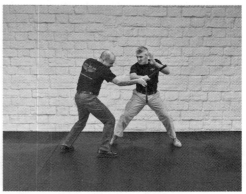

Continue your forward movement past the assailant to counterattack as necessary, keeping your free hand up for protection.

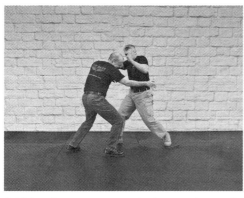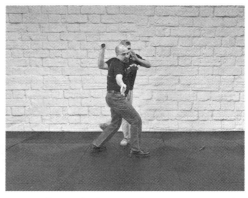

Additional opportune combatives such as a follow-up strike to the head or body may be used.

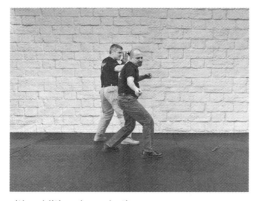

As necessary, continue with additional combatives.

Note: this second preemption option involves the same simultaneous three-part movement as demonstrated in the next defense.

Impact Defense against an Overhead Edged-Weapon Attack

The assailant has the edged weapon in his right hand and is facing you. This attack can involve tremendous force as the assailant presses all of his weight into the attack while using gravity to his advantage. The IKMA curriculum has two defensive options against an overhead or "icepick" type of attack.

Target the weapon arm and then continue your counterattack as necessary. Strive to deflect the edged weapon as close as possible to the assailant's wrist or where a wristwatch would be located. On interception, your impact weapon is positioned to follow a natural strike progression ending with a horizontal strike to the assailant's head.

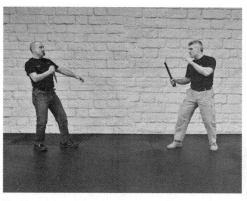 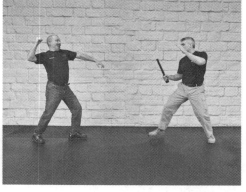

From a right outlet stance and with correct timing, move off the line of attack by stepping diagonally and forward slightly to blade your body. (Note the similarity by design to the previous edged-weapon defense.)

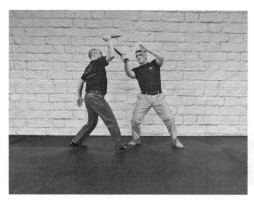 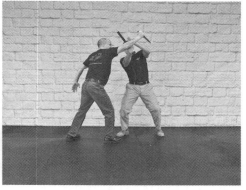

Angle your impact weapon to smash the assailant's knife arm while keeping your free arm up for protection.

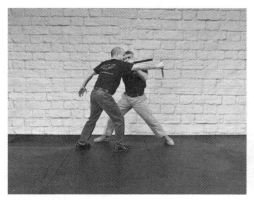 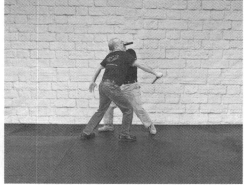

Continue your forward movement past the assailant to counterattack as necessary, using a horizontal backhand strike to the assailant's head while still keeping your free hand up for protection. As an option, you could also seize the attacker's knife arm to control it as you administer additional combatives.

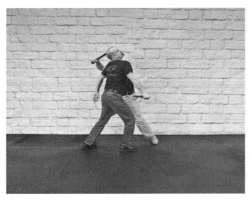 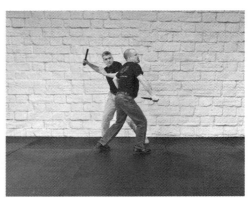

Additional opportune combatives may be used.

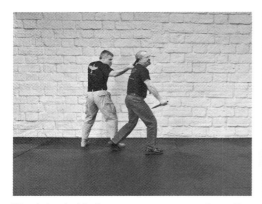 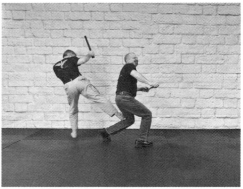

The tai-sabaki step moves you away from the assailant while still keeping him in front of you. As necessary, continue with additional combatives including a low-line side kick.

Impact Defense against an Overhead Edged-Weapon Attack, Variation (Face to Face)

An alternative defense against an overhead stab attack is to step to the outside to move off the line of attack while delivering a strong counter-blow to the assailant's wrist and forearm. In other words, from a right outlet stance (weapon side forward), you step to the outside with your left, which moves your head and torso off the line of attack, while using an outside strike to the assailant's incoming arm.

This alternative defense may be used when

1. you are close to the assailant;
2. you cannot sidestep (such as when you are in close confines or standing against a wall);

3. in a multiple-adversary situation, to keep the defender to the deadside and away from other adversaries; and

4. the assailant comes from an oblique angle (off-angle attack).

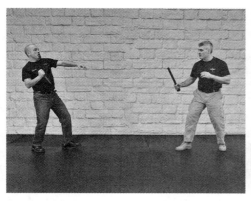 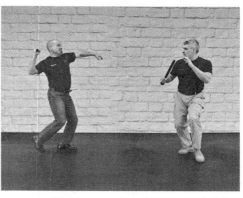

From a right outlet stance and with correct timing, move off the line of attack by stepping diagonally with your rear left leg. (Note the similarity by design to Impact Weapon against Impact Weapon Forehand Side-Swing Attack.)

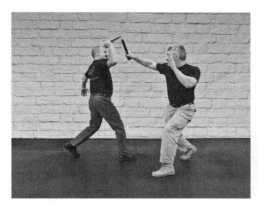 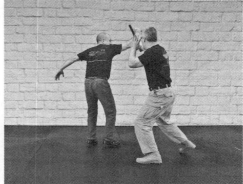

As you continue to step diagonally forward with your left leg, smash the assailant's incoming arm as close to the wrist as fluid targeting will allow. Your impact weapon is positioned to continue with a rotating horizontal strike to the assailant's head or other anatomy as the situation requires. Obviously, even if the assailant dropped the weapon as a result of your initial strike, you may continue with this counterattack method.

Windmill Rotational Defense against an Overhead Edged Weapon (Not Depicted)

You may also use a windmill type of counterattack while retreating, similar to Impact Defenses against an Assailant Posturing with an Edged Weapon (Midlevel).

Outside Impact Defense against a Straight Stab Attack (Not Depicted)

Similar to the outside defense against an overhead stab attack, against a straight stab you may also step to the outside to move off the line of attack while delivering a strong counterblow to the assailant's wrist and forearm. (Your impact weapon is perpendicular to the ground with the tip up.) In other words, from a right outlet stance (weapon side forward), you will step to the outside with your left leg.

This body defense moves your head and torso off the line of attack while using an outside strike to the assailant's incoming arm. Continue to move, switching your stance by withdrawing your right leg (a small tai-sabaki step). At the same time, you deliver additional combatives with the impact weapon. You may close on the assailant using a modified L parry to pin the knife arm to the assailant's torso while you batter him with the impact weapon. This includes hitting his knife hand to dislodge the weapon. Obviously, even if the assailant dropped the weapon as a result of your initial strike, you may continue with this counterattack.

Impact Weapon against an Edged-Weapon Straight Stab, Inside Slash, or Hook Stab

This defense, yet again by design, is nearly identical to Impact Defense against an Overhead Edged-Weapon Attack and can defend against three distinct attacks: straight stab, inside slash, or a hook stab. On interception, your impact weapon is positioned to follow a natural strike progression with a horizontal strike to the assailant's head.

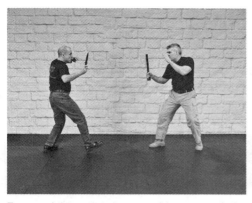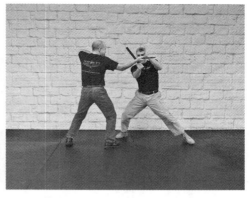

From a right outlet stance, with correct timing, move off the line of attack by stepping diagonally and slightly forward to blade your body. (Note the similarity by design to Impact Weapon against Impact Weapon Forehand Side-Swing Attack.)

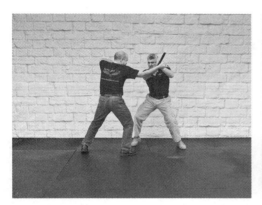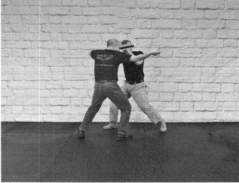

Angle your impact weapon to smash the assailant's knife arm while keeping your free arm up for protection.

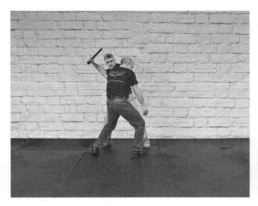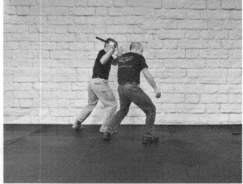

Continue your forward movement past the assailant to counterattack as necessary, using a horizontal backhand strike to the assailant's head while keeping your free hand up for protection.

Impact Defense against a Midlevel Inside Slash

Defending against a midlevel inside slash is similar to defending against a high inside slash, except the defender must invert his impact weapon to better intercept the attacker's incoming knife arm.

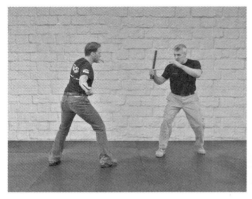
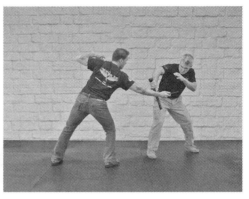

From a right outlet stance, rotate or invert your impact weapon to intercept and smash the assailant's incoming arm.

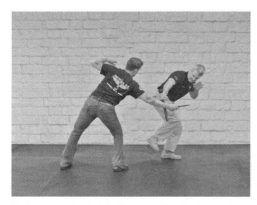
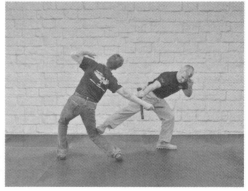

Deliver a side kick to the assailant's forward knee. An alternative is to smash the assailant's arm and then rotate the impact weapon again to hit him in the head. The only danger with this variation is that if the assailant does not drop the weapon, he can slash you as you attempt to hit him in the head.

Impact-Weapon Defense against a Back Slash

This is similar by design to Impact Weapon against Impact Weapon High Backhand Side Swing.

The goal is to burst inside the back slash arc of the edged weapon and jam or smash the assailant's weapon arm with your impact weapon. To close on the assailant, you must switch your stance, keeping your impact weapon perpendicular to the ground. At the same time, your free arm is parallel to your impact weapon to help jam the assailant at the shoulder as he commences the swing. Parry and trap the assailant's arm while executing impact-weapon combatives to his head and weapon arm.

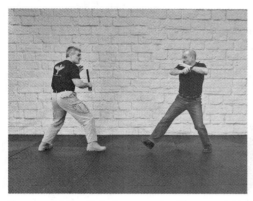 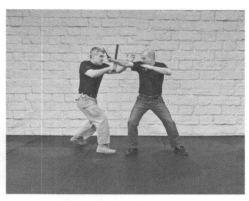

From a right outlet stance and with correct timing, move forward by stepping with both legs on the balls of your feet, keeping your feet equidistant, to intercept his incoming strike. Keep your impact weapon vertical, holding it tightly and strengthening your arm. (Note the similarity by design to Impact Weapon against Impact Weapon High Backhand Side Swing.)

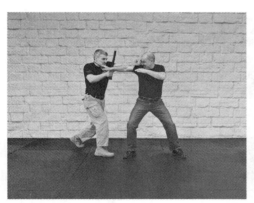 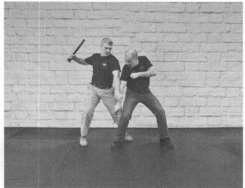

Intercept and smash his incoming arm with your impact weapon. As you intercept his incoming arm, deliver a sliding inverted punch to the assailant's head.

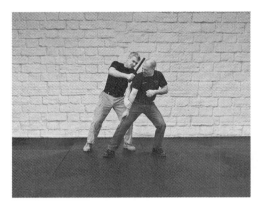 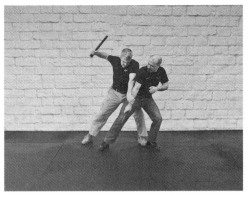

After punching the assailant in the head, use your free hand to clamp down on the assailant's weapon arm, placing your body weight on it to further immobilize it. Continue with additional combatives as necessary.

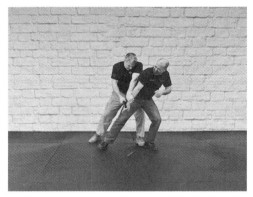

A combative option is to smash the assailant's hand, forcing him to drop the weapon ("defanging the snake").

Windmill Rotational Defense against a Blender Slashing Attack (Not Depicted)

Against an assailant using a blenderlike slashing motion, you may use a continuous outside windmill rotational defense to attack the assailant's head and knife arm. See Impact Defenses against an Assailant Posturing with an Edged Weapon (Midlevel), Windmill Variation. Combine this with a slight retreat. The key is to keep the strong rotation continuous against the assailant's head and knife arm to debilitate him.

Chapter 5

Firearm Cold Combatives

How to Optimize Cold-Weapon Combatives

A combative strike will have optimum force if you accelerate your strike in combination with correct body mechanics. Principally, this involves a total body weight shift through the target. Physics teaches that acceleration times mass equals force. Your strike will generate more force if you accelerate your speed as you extend your arm and put all of your body weight (mass) behind your strike. This requires proper body positioning and technique. Krav maga combatives and techniques do not rely on strength or size. Rather, the system works for anyone regardless of strength or size by emphasizing correct body mechanics. In other words, place all of your body weight behind the strike while rotating with your core strength to connect with the greatest force at maximum speed.

The best way to practice these combatives—as with all techniques—is in stages. Each stage must be isolated, practiced, and perfected. As each stage is mastered it is then combined with the others, creating the whole technique. Using a mirror will help monitor form. While it can be difficult to portray in two-dimensional photos, remember that any combative strike requires the entire body to move in concert.

Regardless of what type of strike you deliver, shifting your body weight forward to deliver your strike will allow you to place all of your body weight behind the strike, connecting with greater force when you combine the strike with maximum speed. Here are some review tips for striking effectively.

Use your entire body. As you strike, move the entire body in concert to use your entire torso. Propelling all of your strength and body weight through the strike will maximize its impact.

Breathe. Exhale as you deliver the strike. Some people like to use a blood-curdling cry as they strike. Either technique—the cry or the exhalation—will prepare your body for both delivering and receiving a strike. Exhaling facilitates oxygen transfer to your muscles, tempers your movements to keep you in control, and creates a vacuum to defend against a counter-strike.

Aim for vulnerable targets. You'll get more for your effort if you strike vulnerable targets. (See "Twenty-Four Vulnerable Targets," chapter 1.)

Here are some of the most common mistakes when attempting both personal- and cold-weapon combatives:

- Making a short movement rather than a long one.
- Pushing the target rather than striking through it.
- Using improper or insufficient weight shift.
- Failing to keep the feet equidistant when stepping.
- Dragging the rear foot rather than pivoting on it.
- Dropping the arm prior to delivering the strike.
- Cocking the arm or winding up.
- Telegraphing the strike by moving the shoulder or head before the hands. The hand should always initiate.
- Stutter-stepping or dropping the arms while "winding up" to deliver a kick.
- Dropping the other arm or both arms.
- Failing to recover immediately into a fighting stance.
- Failing to breathe correctly.
- For rear elbow strikes, failing to pivot the front foot, which must move slightly to accommodate the full follow-through.
- Failing to pivot correctly (that is, on the ball of the foot, which allows the base leg to turn 90 degrees).
- Kicking straight with the knee on an angle, sending the kick off course and also delivering less power.
- Launching a kick improperly by "chambering" it or bringing the knee up to deliver a snap kick, rather than coming from "below the radar."
- Hunching over rather than standing tall with the kick.

- Delivering a front kick with the toes or the heel rather than the ball of the foot.

- Dropping the arms prior to delivering the kick or while launching the kick.

- Bending the kicking leg too much on impact. A slight bend is OK to prevent hyperextension.

- Failing to roll the hip over for a roundhouse kick. The kick then resembles a poor inside slap kick.

Mastering Personal, Impact, and Firearm Combined Combatives

Many people think of hand-to-hand combat as exactly that: primarily using one's hands. Yet correct krav maga incorporates upper-body, lower-body, and cold-weapon combatives in simultaneous combinations. In other words, clubbing, slashing, thrusting, kicks, punches, eye gouges or whips, elbows, and knees are all combined for an overwhelming counterattack; the weapon is not used exclusively. A weapon—either one of opportunity or a designated one—should be considered simply an extension of the body.

Cold-weapon combatives, in many ways, are slight modifications of open-handed combatives. Hence, the importance of learning krav maga's core combative movements, which readily translate into cold-weapon capabilities. This building combative methodology is one of the reasons krav maga is so popular and why elements of the system have been adopted by militaries and law enforcement agencies all over the world.

Low-Line Kick Emphasis

Krav maga emphasizes low-line kicks. In developing its self-defense close-quarters-combat program, the IDF forced its soldiers to run long distances with full combat loads. Many of these test candidates were accomplished martial artists who favored high kicks to the head. After an exhausting run in full "battle rattle," the candidates were told to defend against an attack using whatever techniques they felt most comfortable using. Few of the candidates skilled in high kicks could perform them. Their physical taxation prior to the fighting tests made it extremely difficult to kick high. The IDF recognized the need to use only self-defense close-quarters-combat techniques that would work for all trainees, especially under trying circumstances. Therefore, low kicks combined with upper body combatives became integral to krav maga training and more difficult to defend.

Cold-Weapon Retzev

As noted, you can combine cold-weapon strikes with hand and elbow strikes (when working with impact weapons, edged weapons, or handguns) and kicks. Withdraw your striking arm(s) quickly into your fighting stance to maintain your defensive and offensive capabilities. As soon as you land the front strike and are retracting your arm, launch the rear strike. The momentum of drawing the front strike back will help catapult the rear strike forward, creating more impact. Our curriculum has a specific program for integrating cold-weapon combatives with personal combatives.

The following combatives are shown for cold weapons but use the same basic mechanics as a hand strike. Krav maga's underlying strategy is to show one core movement with variations or accommodations. In other words, the footwork, pivoting, and weight-transfer dynamics all remain the same for all thrusting, horizontal, diagonal, or uppercut open-handed strikes.

Handgun Straight Thrust

When using this direct and fast strike, aim for the face, jaw, or throat. You can also aim at the solar plexus or stomach. The correct body mechanics for this strike are similar to those in a baton straight thrust, handgun, or long gun: the body must work in concert as you pivot through the thrust, transferring your entire weight and moving your feet correctly. The idea, as with all combatives, is to refine your body's natural motion.

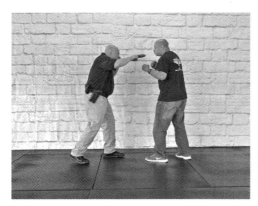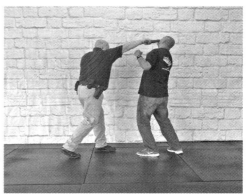

From a left outlet stance gripping the handgun securely, pivot on the ball of your right foot while simultaneously extending your right arm, thrusting the weapon's muzzle into your target. As your arm extends to deliver the strike, tighten your grip. Make contact with your hand parallel to the ground. Raise your right shoulder slightly while tucking your chin into it to protect your jaw and neck.

Handgun Three-Point Strike

This quick handgun strike variation presents three sharp edges of the weapon: the muzzle, trigger guard, and magazine.

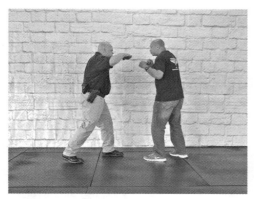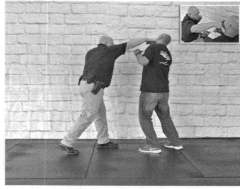

From a left outlet stance gripping the handgun securely, pivot on the ball of your right foot while simultaneously extending your right arm, thrusting the weapon's muzzle into your target. As your arm extends to deliver the strike, tighten your grip. Make contact with your hand parallel to the ground. Raise your right shoulder slightly while tucking your chin into it to protect your jaw and neck. Continue with additional retzev combatives as necessary.

Handgun Half-Roundhouse Strike

When using this powerful, slightly off-angle strike, aim for the nose, jaw, or throat. You will attack your adversary with tremendous force using the muzzle of the weapon. This strike differs from the straight strike because the arm does not shoot out directly toward the target, but rather uses a slight angle of attack.

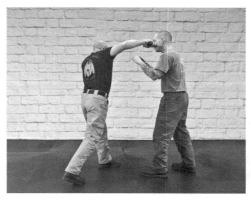

From a left outlet stance grip the handgun securely and pivot on the ball of your right foot while simultaneously extending your right arm, thrusting the weapon's muzzle off angle into your target.

As your arm extends to deliver the strike, tighten your grip. Make contact with your hand parallel to the ground. Raise your right shoulder slightly while tucking your chin into it to protect your jaw and neck. To facilitate the off-angle strike, the right side of your body will pivot into the strike while your nonstriking shoulder will angle slightly away. Continue with additional retzev combatives as necessary.

Long-Gun Straight Muzzle Thrust

A long-gun muzzle thrust is a highly effective combative. Optimum targets are the face and throat. To be sure, linear movements such as a straight thrust are easiest for an operator who is heavily laden with body armor and equipment.

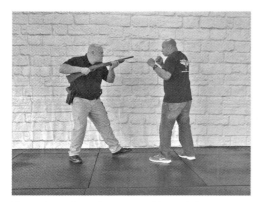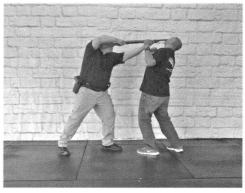

From the left outlet stance (for a right-handed shooter), initiate the thrust with the left leg stepping forward, accelerating the weapon as your right leg steps forward the same distance. The thrust is naturally followed by additional combatives, including a horizontal or uppercut butt strike, or forward slash with the barrel. Aim for vulnerable anatomy such as the face, throat, solar plexus, or groin, depending on your height. Continue with additional retzev combatives as necessary.

Long-Gun Magazine Strike

A long-gun magazine thrust is another highly effective combative. When using this short, direct, and rapid strike, aim for the throat, jaw, or nose. With your body weight behind it and with proper footwork, this technique is extremely powerful for knocking your adversary back, especially if you strike the throat. Once again, linear movements such as a straight thrust are easiest for an operator who is heavily laden with body armor and equipment. Further note that the magazine thrust is naturally followed by additional combatives, including a horizontal or uppercut butt strike, or forward slash with the barrel.

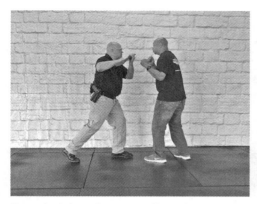 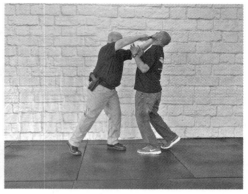

From the left outlet stance (for a right-handed shooter), initiate the thrust with the left leg stepping forward, accelerating the weapon forward as your right leg steps forward the same distance. Thrust your arms as you transfer your weight and pivot slightly with your rear right foot. Continue with additional retzev combatives as necessary.

Handgun "Body Shot" Strikes

This strike, by simple design, is similar to a straight thrust to the head. This tactic can damage the adversary's groin area or knock the wind out of him. Obviously, if delivered with enough force and accuracy, it can break an adversary's ribs and damage internal organs. As with all combatives, pivot correctly on the balls of your feet, driving the handgun's barrel through the adversary.

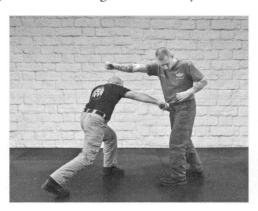 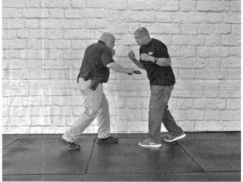

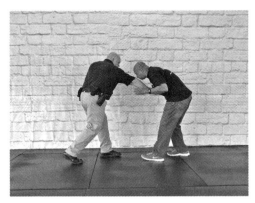

From a left outlet stance, gripping the handgun securely, pivot on the ball of your right foot while extending your right arm, thrusting the weapon's muzzle into your target. As your arm extends to deliver the strike, tighten your grip. Raise your right shoulder slightly while tucking your chin to protect your jaw and neck. The upper- and lower-body movements are similar to those of the right rear straight thrust. Continue with additional retzev combatives as necessary.

Handgun Inward Chop

The strike's path follows whatever opening your adversary gives you. Optimum targets include the jaw, cheek, throat, ear, and temple but may also include the body, as noted below.

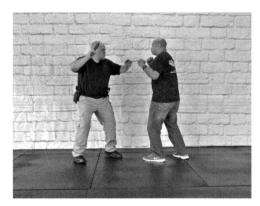
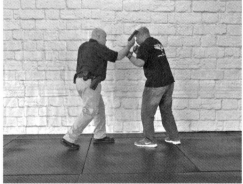

Begin in your regular outlet stance with your hands protecting your face. Bend your elbow anywhere from 60 to 90 degrees, again, depending on the angle of attack you choose. As you deliver the inward chop, pivot on your rear foot in the same direction as the strike.

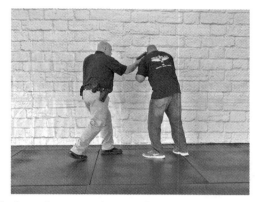

As you pivot on the ball of your foot, turn the rest of your body, but keep your eyes on the target. Adjust your front foot slightly to accommodate your rear foot's movement. Keep your rear hand up in a fighting position. Continue with additional retzev combatives as necessary.

Horizontal Long-Gun Butt Strikes

Provided you are not wearing a restrictive sling, this powerful strike's path follows whatever opening your adversary gives you. Optimum targets include the jaw, cheek, throat, and ear.

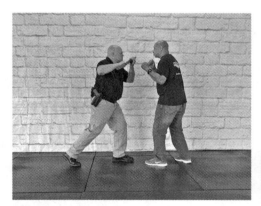
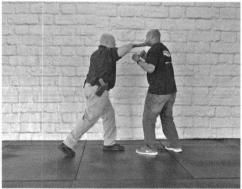

From the left outlet stance, pivot on the ball of your rear foot to deliver the strike through the target. The upper-body or rifle-butt movement precedes the lower-body movement by a fraction of a second. Use the weapon's stock, not your elbow, to make impact.

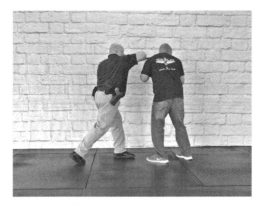

To accommodate the rear foot pivot, the ball of your front foot should pivot slightly as well. Note: for modern assault rifles using pistol grips, be sure to angle the butt outward. Continue with additional retzev combatives as necessary.

Outward Handgun Chop

This technique best targets the sides of the neck (carotid arteries), throat, and temple, using the underside of the barrel. The outward handgun chop uses the underside of the barrel as the inward handgun chop; however, the wrist rotates to position the handgun's grip to the outside.

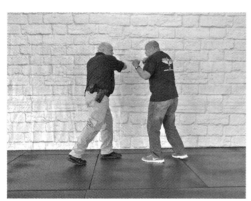 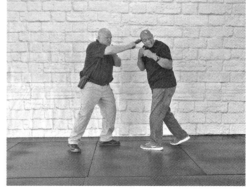

As you close on the assailant, open your hips in the direction of your strike and begin to spin your body toward your adversary, leading with the weapon arm. As your body spins and your hips open up, your striking weapon arm swings around. As you deliver the handgun outward chop, hit with the underside of the barrel. Keep your elbow joint slightly bent to avoid any hyper-extension on impact. Pivot slightly on the balls of both feet in the same direction as the chop so that your toes turn past the target. As you pivot on the balls of your feet, turn the rest of your body, but keep your eyes on the target. Adjust your rear foot slightly to accommodate your front foot's movement. Keep your rear hand up in a fighting position. Continue with additional retzev combatives as necessary.

Long-Gun Slash

Similar to the outward handgun chop, the long-gun slash targets the head, temple, ear, sides of the neck (carotid arteries), and throat, using the underside of the barrel.

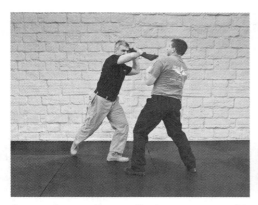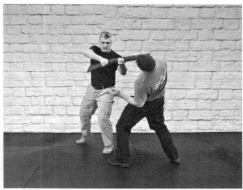

As you close on the assailant, open up your hips in the direction of your strike and begin to spin your body toward your adversary, leading with the weapon arm. As your body spins and your hips open up, your forward arm swings around, delivering the strike with the underside of the barrel. Pivot the front foot in the same direction as the slash so that your toes turn past the target. As you pivot on the ball of your foot, turn the rest of your body, but keep your eyes on the target. Adjust your rear foot slightly to accommodate your front foot's movement. Keep your rear hand up in a fighting position. Natural follow-up strikes include a horizontal butt strike or uppercut butt strike. Continue with additional retzev combatives as necessary.

Over-the-Top Long-Gun Butt Strike

The over-the-top long-gun butt strike is designed to slam down on your adversary and is somewhat similar to the hammer strike. Targets include the eye ridge, nose, ear, and throat. For the handgun, the weapon's barrel rakes down on the target. Be sure to pivot on the balls of your feet for maximum power.

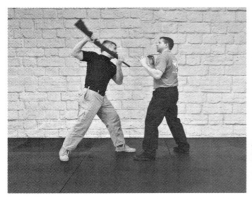
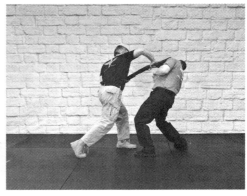

From the left outlet stance, rotate the long gun up and then over to slam down on the target. Again, pivot on the balls of your feet to engage your hips and core for maximum power. The over-the-top strike uses a hip pivot movement that is a compromise between the movements used in the straight strike and the roundhouse strike. Your arms should not cross but move parallel to one another. Continue with additional retzev combatives as necessary.

Long-Gun Uppercut Strikes

The uppercut strike can seriously damage your adversary's exposed chin, throat, or groin (when you are on the ground and your adversary is standing). Note: a common mistake is to drop the long-gun arm rather than the body. This does not harness the power of the hips. In making this mistake, this type of strike has minimal power and can be easily defended.

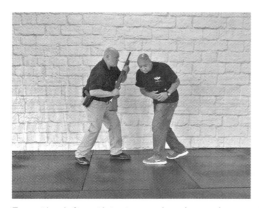
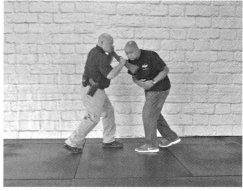

From the left outlet stance, bend your knees slightly to generate power from the lower body, allowing your hips to explode through the target. Pivot the front leg inward and straighten your knees as you strike, delivering an upward blow from across your body. The arms should move naturally in concert; do not cross them.

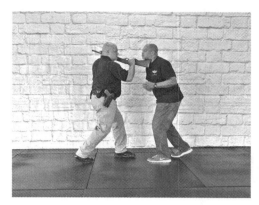

Be sure to pivot on the rear foot for maximum power to explode with the hips through the target. A natural follow-up strike is a long-gun slash. Continue with additional retzev combatives as necessary. For modern assault rifles with pistol grips, be sure to angle the butt outward.

Long-Gun Hammer-Type Vertical Drop Strikes

This hammer-type strike smashes down on the adversary using your body weight momentum combined with the weapon's heft. Note: a similar strike could be used with a handgun, striking with the barrel or possibly with the grip, but this may cause the magazine to dislodge.

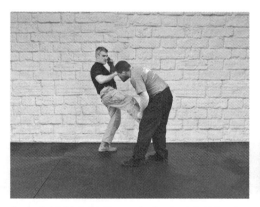
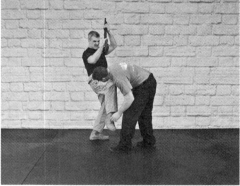

A straight kick to the groin is depicted to show how the assailant's body would double over to expose the back of the neck or head.

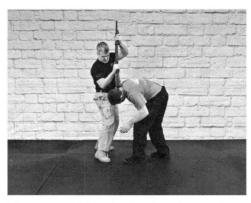

If possible, deliver the strike as your kicking leg touches down, using your body weight to maximize the strike's power. Continue with additional retzev combatives as necessary.

Rear Horizontal Long-Gun Butt Strikes

The perpendicular long-gun butt strike is a compact strike to a threat from the rear. It targets the adversary's face, throat, or solar plexus. Your hips once again create the power by opening up as you take a short step backward with the leg on the same side.

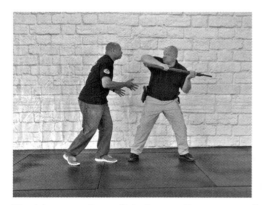 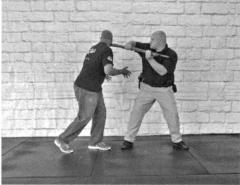

Start in a regular outlet stance. Keep your striking arm close to your body and look over your shoulder in the direction of your strike. Step back slightly with the leg on the butt side of the long gun. As you shift your body weight through the strike, make impact with the long-gun butt to the face, throat, or solar plexus. Continue with additional retzev combatives as necessary.

Rear Low Long-Gun Butt Strikes

Similar to the rear horizontal butt strike, the rear low long-gun butt strike delivers a compact strike to a rear threat, targeting the adversary's midsection or groin. In this long-gun strike, your hips once again create the power by opening up with the same-side leg.

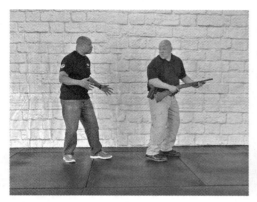 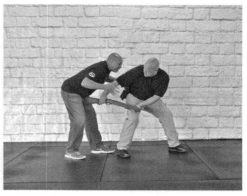

Start in a regular outlet stance. Keeping your striking arm close to your body, look over your shoulder in the direction of your strike. Step back slightly with the leg on the butt side of the long gun. As you shift your body weight through the strike, drive the long-gun butt into the adversary's groin, stomach, solar plexus, throat, or face. Continue with retzev combatives as necessary.

Rear Vertical Long-Gun Butt Strike

This strike is a natural follow-on to the rear low long-gun butt strike, which doubles an adversary over. The rear vertical long-gun butt strike involves exploding upward with your hips, shoulder, and arm, targeting the solar plexus, throat, or face with the end of the long-gun butt.

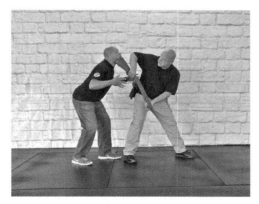

Keeping your rear arm close to your body with your body coiled by bending your knees, look over your shoulder in the direction of your strike. Explode with the rifle butt through your adversary's chin. Continue with retzev combatives as necessary.

Long-Gun Cold Weapons against Personal and Cold Weapons

Long-gun defenses against impact- and edged-weapon attacks are, once again by design, nearly identical. In addition, the long defenses somewhat mimic some of the shorter impact-weapon defenses against impact and edged weapons examined previously. Again, krav maga emphasizes one core tactic to defeat multiple attack and variable weapon scenarios.

With the advent of twenty-first-century weaponry, some krav maga defenses have necessarily been modified. When Imi first developed the long-gun defenses, the IDF generally used Mauser Kar 98K and Lee-Enfield variants. These rifles, even the carbine versions, were relatively long. In addition, a soldier could wield the rifle like a short staff. The IDF then began to adopt the FN FAL, a very long rifle with a pistol grip, and the Uzi submachine gun, a compact weapon. In addition, select IDF units used captured Kalashnikov assault rifle variants. When using these firearms, soldiers had to adapt krav maga techniques to suit the weapon.

The long barrel of the FAL could be used effectively to slash and thrust along with parrying an enemy's hand-to-hand attack. The IDF replaced the FAL with the Galil family of rifles and subsequently incorporated the M-16/4 series. The most current 5.56 small arm the IDF has adopted is the Tavor bull-pup family design. Krav maga long-gun defenses are also adapted for long guns with pistol-like vertical foregrips or shortened barrels. For the modern operator, a foregrip substantially modifies his parrying and deflection capability. Shorter barrels, used in urban settings, also modify a defender's deflection capabilities.

Some of the defenses, where applicable, will be shown with two different long guns and how each respective design or configuration and grip may require the defense to be modified. Due to varying weapon lengths, configurations, and designs, the principles involved in defending with long guns must be absorbed and applied rather than the specifics for each weapon category depicted.

Note: the following defenses assume your long gun is inoperable, you are caught by surprise or ambushed while in the negative five, or you wish to use a cold-weapon lesser force option. These defenses are depicted with the long gun in the low ready rifle position, as this is the position most commonly used. A long-gun high ready position has advantages in that it makes the more common high attack line defenses easier but low attack line defenses more difficult. So, you must adapt. Importantly, the high ready rifle position would modify a few of the defenses. Where applicable, this change is noted. Obviously, regardless of assuming a low or high ready rifle position, shooting the assailant before he attacks you is your first option.

Note: for each of the following long-gun examples, after defending against the threat with the long gun, the defender should create distance and bring the weapon back on line or "back into battery" with a clear field of fire. In the alternative, if more expedient, the defender should create distance to deploy a secondary weapon.

Long Gun against a Straight Punch

If your long gun is inoperable or out of ammunition and an assailant is foolhardy enough to attempt a straight punch against you, use the long gun as an impact weapon. Combine intercepting and attacking his incoming arm with a body defense. Sidestep his punch and move to his deadside.

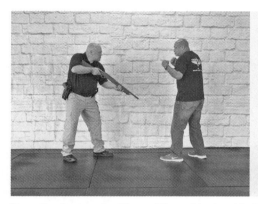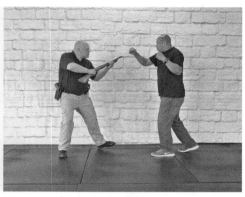

From the low ready rifle position, sidestep his incoming straight punch by stepping diagonally with your left foot, followed by your right foot. As you step, use the long gun to intercept and deflect his incoming arm. Note: depending on standard tactics, techniques, and procedures (TTPs), if the long gun is held in the high ready rifle position, this defense becomes even easier.

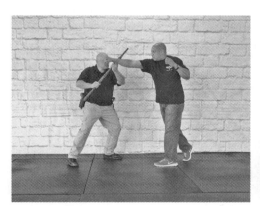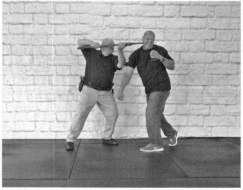

As you batter the extended arm, immediately transition to a straight thrust to the assailant's head. Continue with additional retzev combatives as necessary.

Inoperable Long Gun against a Hook Punch

If your long gun is inoperable or you have use-of-force considerations against an assailant who is foolish enough to attempt a straight punch against you, use the long gun's length in a direct thrust at the assailant's vulnerable anatomy. Another alternative is to use the long gun as an impact weapon combined with a body defense to sidestep his incoming punch and move to his deadside. At the same time, you intercept and attack his incoming arm. After battering the assailant's punching arm, use the barrel of the weapon to slash at the assailant's head.

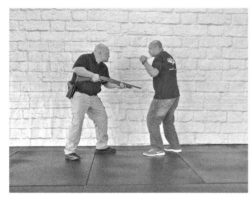 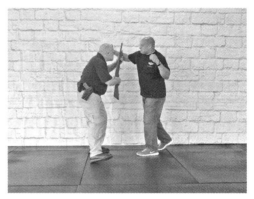

From the ready position, as you recognize his incoming hook punch, sidestep the punch by stepping diagonally with your right foot, followed by your left foot. As you step, use the long gun to intercept his incoming arm. Note: once again, depending on standard tactics, techniques, and procedures (TTPs), if the long gun is held in the high ready rifle position, this defense becomes even easier.

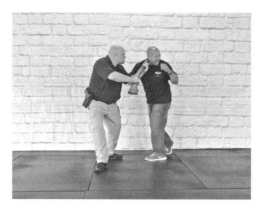

As you batter the extended arm, immediately transition to a slash to the assailant's head or neck. Natural follow-on strikes include horizontal or uppercut butt strikes (provided a sling will allow these combatives). Continue with additional retzev combatives as necessary or create distance to render the long gun operable or deploy a secondary weapon.

Inoperable Long Gun Thrust against a Tackle

If your long gun is inoperable or out of ammunition and an assailant is foolhardy enough to attempt to tackle you, use the long gun as an impact weapon. Another alternative is to use the long gun as an impact weapon combined with a body defense to sidestep his incoming tackle and move to his deadside. At the same time, you intercept and attack the opponent's lowered head as he drops for the tackle attempt. You may then use the barrel of the weapon to slash at the back of the assailant's head.

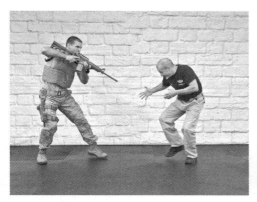 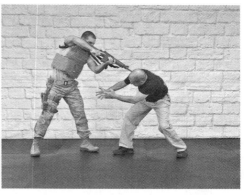

From the ready position, as the assailant lowers his level to attempt the tackle, thrust the muzzle into his head. If you recognize the attack soon enough, you may also step off the line of attack as you thrust the muzzle into the side of his face or head from an off angle.

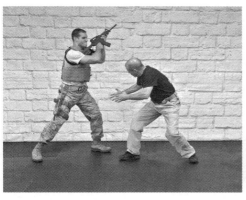 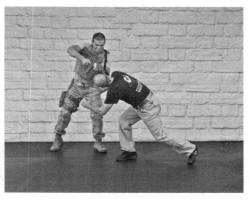

As you jolt the head of the assailant, you can—if necessary—slash down on the assailant's head.

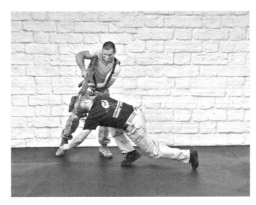

Natural follow-on strikes include horizontal or uppercut butt strikes (provided a sling will allow these combatives). Continue with additional retzev combatives as necessary.

Long-Gun Thrust with Sidestep against a Tackle

If an assailant is reckless enough to attempt a tackle against you when your long gun is inoperable or out of ammunition, or if you wish to use a lesser force cold-weapon option, use the weapon's length in a direct thrust at the assailant's vulnerable anatomy. Another alternative is to use the long gun as an impact weapon combined with a body defense to sidestep his incoming tackle and move to his deadside. At the same time, you intercept and attack the opponent's lowered head as he drops for the tackle attempt. You then use the barrel of the weapon to slash at the back of the assailant's head.

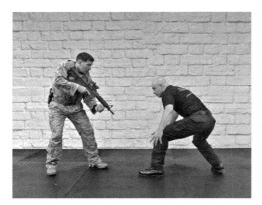
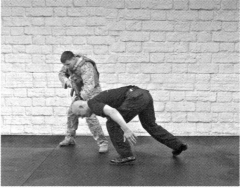

From the low ready rifle position, if you recognize the attack soon enough, you may step off the line of attack as you thrust the muzzle into the side of his face or head from an off angle. Natural follow-on strikes include horizontal or uppercut butt strikes (provided a sling will allow these combatives). Continue with additional retzev combatives as necessary.

Long-Gun Defense against an Overhead Impact-Weapon Attack

The IKMA curriculum has two defensive options against an overhead impact attack when your long gun is inoperable. Notably, these impact-weapon defenses would also work against a machete attack (depicted next). The parrying defense is designed to protect the defender's forward hand gripping the weapon.

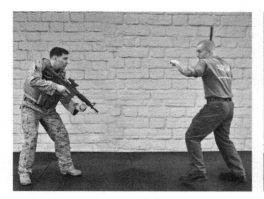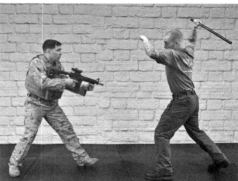

From the low ready rifle position, raise the long gun and close on the assailant.

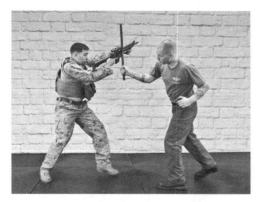

Intercept his incoming overhead attack, angling the long gun slightly on impact to make the weapon slide off.

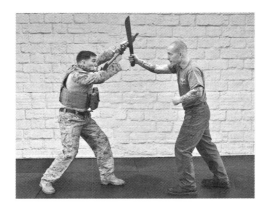

A machete variation is depicted and defended the same as an overhead impact defense.

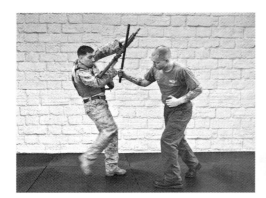
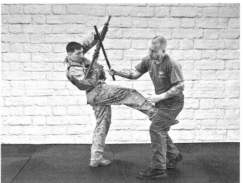

As you intercept the overhead strike, kick the assailant in the groin (the front or rear leg may be used). Natural follow-on strikes include horizontal or uppercut butt strikes (provided a sling will allow these combatives). Continue with additional retzev combatives as necessary.

Long-Gun Defense against an Overhead Machete Attack, Sidestep and Parry

This variation from the low ready rifle position allows the defender to sidestep the overhead attack and move to the assailant's deadside. This same defense could be used against an overhead impact weapon. The assailant has a machete in his right hand and is facing you.

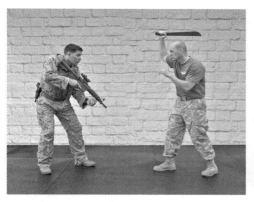 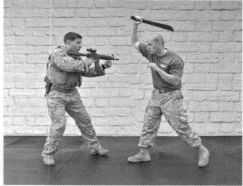

From the low ready rifle position, raise the long gun and close on the assailant by sidestepping forward diagonally.

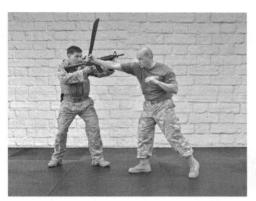 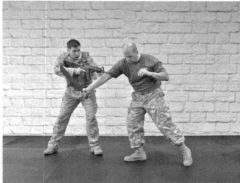

Intercept his incoming overhead attack with the long gun slightly angled to allow the machete to slip off. Keep moving to the assailant's deadside.

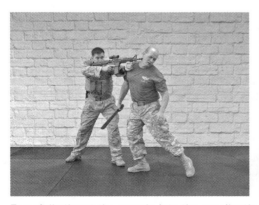 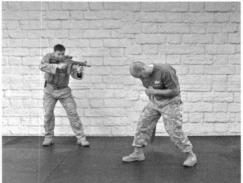

Forcefully thrust the muzzle into the assailant's head or face. Natural follow-on strikes include horizontal or uppercut butt strikes (provided a sling will allow these combatives). Continue with additional retzev combatives as necessary or create distance, giving yourself the opportunity to render the firearm operable.

Long-Gun Preemptive Thrust Defense against an Overhead Edged-Weapon Attack

The IKMA curriculum has two defensive options against an overhead or "icepick" type of attack when your long gun is inoperable:

1.   an intercepting thrust
2.   a sidestep and simultaneous counterattack

Use your long gun's length to intercept the assailant before he can lunge forward with the knife. A straight thrust to the assailant's solar plexus, throat, or face is highly effective in initially halting the attack. The thrust relies heavily on timing and is difficult if you are using a bull-pup or short SMG-designed weapon. To execute the defense properly, you must extend the long gun at the correct time and with considerable accuracy to damage the assailant before his overhead attacking arm comes forward.

After thwarting the initial attack, continue with counterattacks, including additional long-gun combatives and a straight kick to the groin or side kick to the knee. You may move to the assailant's knife-arm side, immediately slashing at the arm to break it or at least make him drop the weapon. If the assailant folds back, you may also go to the other side to stay away from the knife arm. The follow-up, as with all defenses, is dependent on how the assailant is affected by your initial combative.

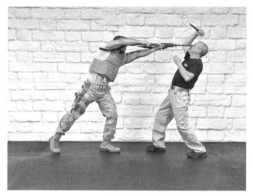

Recognize the assailant's grip of the edged weapon and, therefore, how it might be employed. Thrust the muzzle straight into the assailant's face or throat. Continue with retzev combatives to disable the assailant, including smashing his knife-wielding arm to force him to drop the weapon. Of course, if the long gun is inoperable, render it functional or use a secondary weapon to shoot the assailant (as necessary and justified).

Long-Gun Outside Defense against an Overhead Edged-Weapon Attack

This defense batters the assailant's arm as it descends toward you while taking you to the deadside. Strive to deflect the edged weapon as close as possible to the assailant's wrist or where a wristwatch would be located.

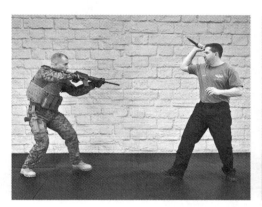 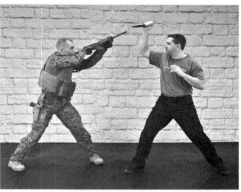

Recognize the assailant's grip of the edged weapon and, therefore, how it might be employed. From the low ready rifle position, raise the long gun and close on the assailant by sidestepping forward diagonally. Note: from a high ready rifle position this defense is that much more direct by having the barrel already in position to deflect and counterattack.

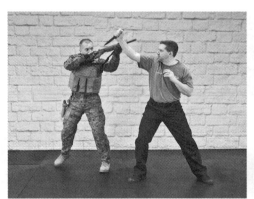 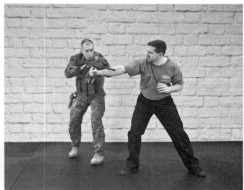

Intercept his incoming overhead attack, angling the long gun slightly to hit with the barrel and allowing the knife arm to slide off and away while you keep moving forward to the assailant's deadside.

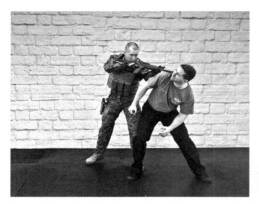 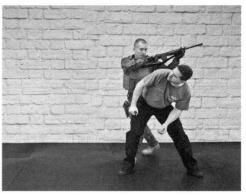

After deflecting his incoming strike, immediately thrust the muzzle into the assailant's head or face. Keep moving to the assailant's deadside. Natural follow-on strikes include horizontal or uppercut butt strikes (provided a sling will allow these combatives).

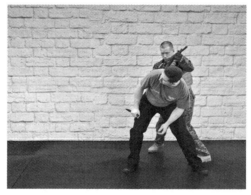

Continue with additional retzev combatives as necessary or create distance, allowing you the opportunity to render the firearm operable.

We present two long-gun defenses against an overhead edged-weapon attack. For either defensive option, the defender stands in a left outlet stance (assuming he shoots right handed). As with the previous impact-weapon defenses, either variation requires the defender to step off the line, attack the incoming knife arm, and continue with retzev counterattacks to neutralize the threat.

Long-Gun Outside Defense against an Overhead Edged-Weapon Attack

This variation from the low ready rifle position focuses on using a shorter-barreled weapon with a "broomstick" foregrip and short sling. Be aware that the short sling may limit the long gun's strike capabilities as a cold weapon. Once again, strive to deflect the edged weapon as close as possible to the assailant's wrist or where a wristwatch would be located.

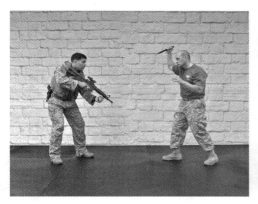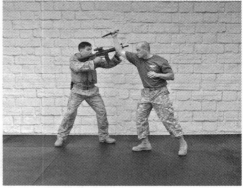

Recognize the assailant's grip of the edged weapon and, therefore, how it might be employed. From the low ready rifle position, raise the long gun and close on the assailant by sidestepping forward diagonally. Note: once again, if your TTPs call for a high ready rifle position, the defense becomes that much easier.

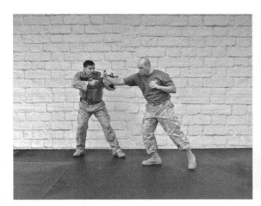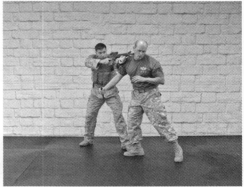

Intercept his incoming overhead attack, angling the long gun slightly to hit with the barrel and allowing the knife arm to slide off and away. Immediately thrust the muzzle into the assailant's head or face. Keep moving to his deadside. Natural follow-on strikes include horizontal or uppercut butt strikes (provided a sling will allow these combatives). Continue with additional retzev combatives as necessary or create distance, allowing you to render the firearm operable.

The IKMA curriculum does not advocate a direct block of an overhead stab since the defender still remains on the line of attack. This is especially perilous with modern bull-pup long-gun designs. In addition, the assailant can snag the long gun with his knife, possibly lowering the defender's defense while the assailant has a free arm to initiate another attack. In any event, whether you stand still and absorb the full impact of his incoming arm or, preferably, step off the line with two hands on the long gun, be sure to deliver a simultaneous or near-simultaneous kick in keeping with krav maga's principles of combined defense and attack.

Submachine-Gun Outside Defense against an Overhead Edged-Weapon Attack

This variation focuses on using a submachine gun. The mechanics are the same as shown in previous defense; however, the defender must adjust for the short length of the submachine gun. Once again, strive to deflect the edged weapon as close as possible to the assailant's wrist or where a wristwatch would be located.

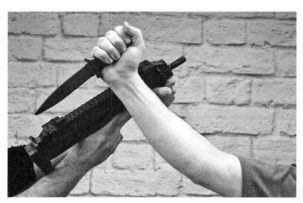

Recognize the assailant's grip of the edged weapon and, therefore, how it might be employed. Deflect his incoming overhead strike by rotating the submachine gun to use its length to parry the attack. Continue with additional retzev combatives or create distance to bring the weapon or another online.

Long Gun (Short-Sling Variation) against an Edged-Weapon Hook Stab (Face to Face)

This defense is represented using a short sling so the weapon cannot be maneuvered freely.

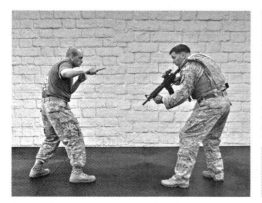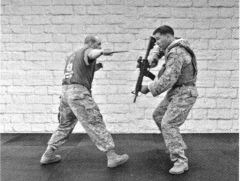

Recognize the assailant's grip of the edged weapon and, therefore, how it might be employed. From the low ready rifle position, pointing the muzzle to the ground, keep the weapon's length perpendicular as you burst into the assailant. From a high ready rifle position this defense would change similar to the defense depicted in Long-Gun Defense against a Forward Slash.

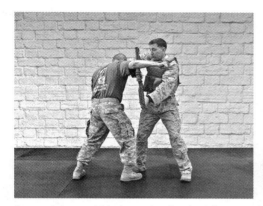 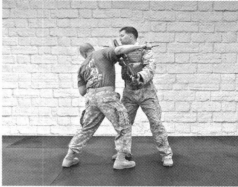

As you intercept his incoming hook stab, use a lateral elbow strike against the assailant's head.

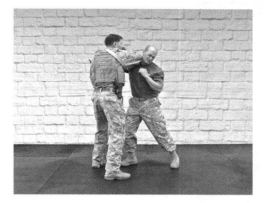

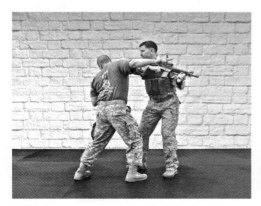 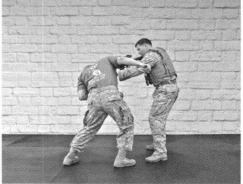

Continue your counterattack, bringing the weapon to bear as a cold weapon.

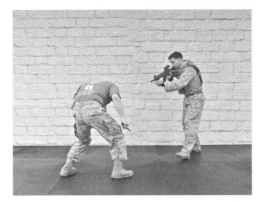

Continue with additional retzev combatives as necessary or create distance and give yourself an opportunity to render your long gun operable.

Long Gun against a Straight Edged-Weapon Stab

By design, this defense against a straight stab is nearly identical to Long-Gun Outside Defense against an Overhead Edged-Weapon Attack.

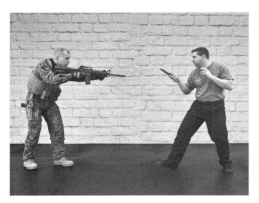 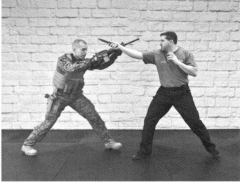

Recognize the assailant's grip of the edged weapon and, therefore, how it might be employed. From the ready position, raise the long gun and close on the assailant by sidestepping forward diagonally. Intercept his straight stab, angling the long gun slightly to hit with the barrel and allowing his knife arm to slide down and away as you keep moving forward to the assailant's deadside.

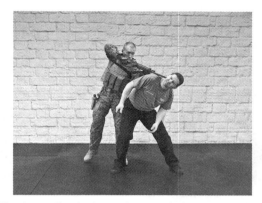

After deflecting his strike, immediately thrust the muzzle into the assailant's head or face. Keep moving to the assailant's deadside. Natural follow-on strikes include horizontal or uppercut butt strikes (provided a sling will allow these combatives). Continue with additional retzev combatives as necessary or create distance to render the firearm operable.

Long Gun (Short Barrel) against a Straight Edged-Weapon Stab

By design, this defense from the low ready rifle position against a straight stab with an inoperable long gun is nearly identical to Long-Gun Outside Defense against an Overhead Edged-Weapon Attack.

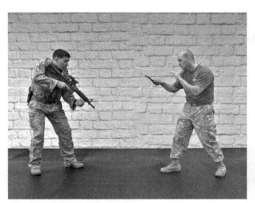 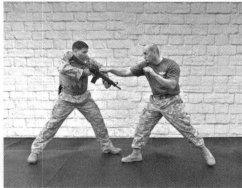

Recognize the assailant's grip of the edged weapon and, therefore, how it might be employed. From the low ready rifle position, raise the long gun and close on the assailant by sidestepping forward diagonally. Rotate the long gun down, angling it to use its length (topside) to intercept his straight stab. Note: from a high ready position the defense would be similar Long Gun against a Straight Edged-Weapon Back Slash (Face to Face).

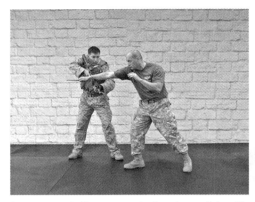 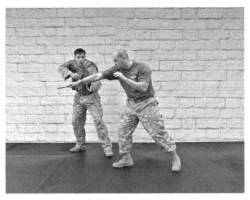

Smash the knife arm and allow it to slide off and away from the barrel while you keep moving forward to the assailant's deadside.

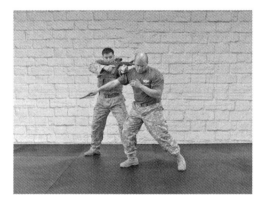

After deflecting his incoming strike, immediately thrust the muzzle into the assailant's head or face. Keep moving to the assailant's deadside. Natural follow-on strikes include horizontal or uppercut butt strikes (provided a sling will allow these combatives). Continue with additional retzev combatives as necessary or create distance to render the firearm once again operable.

Long Gun (Short Barrel) against a Machete Straight Stab

By design, this defense against a machete straight stab is nearly identical to Long Gun against a Straight Edged-Weapon Stab. It is appropriate when the defender has an inoperable long gun.

From the low ready rifle position, raise the long gun and close on the assailant by sidestepping forward diagonally. Intercept his incoming straight stab attack, angling the long gun slightly to deflect below the ACOG® sight and allow the knife arm to deflect off and away while you keep moving forward to the assailant's deadside. After deflecting the assailant's incoming strike, immediately thrust the muzzle into his head or face. Keep moving to his deadside. Natural follow-on strikes include horizontal or uppercut butt strikes, provided a sling will allow these combatives. Continue with additional retzev combatives as necessary or create distance to render the firearm once again operable.

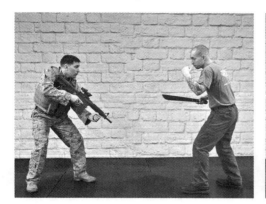 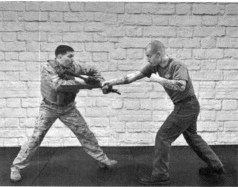

From the low ready rifle position, raise the long gun and close on the assailant by sidestepping forward diagonally. Rotate the long gun down, angling it to use its length (topside) to intercept his straight stab.

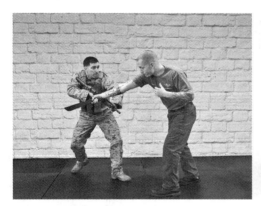 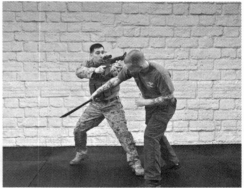

Smash the knife arm and allow it to slide along the barrel while you keep moving forward to the assailant's deadside. After deflecting his incoming strike, immediately thrust the muzzle into the assailant's head or face. Keep moving to the assailant's deadside. Natural follow-on strikes include horizontal or uppercut butt strikes (provided a sling will allow these combatives). Continue with additional retzev combatives as necessary or create distance to render the firearm once again operable.

Submachine Gun against a Straight Edged-Weapon Stab

By design, this defense with an inoperable SMG is nearly identical to Long Gun against a Straight Edged-Weapon Stab.

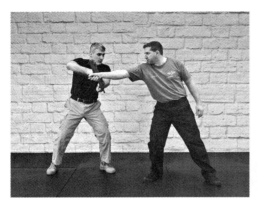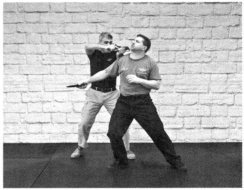

Smash the knife arm and allow it to slide off and away from the barrel while you keep moving forward to the assailant's deadside.

Long-Gun Defenses against a Low Edged Stab

The IKMA curriculum has two defensive options with an inoperable long-gun against an underhand stab:

1. an intercepting thrust
2. a sidestep and simultaneous counterattack

When defending against a low straight stab, the preemptive long-gun thrust is particularly effective. You may use the long gun's length to smash the assailant in the face before he can reach you with the edged weapon.

You are in a left outlet stance with the long gun in ready-parry position or an "on-guard" stance. Using timing to preempt the rise of the stabbing arm, the defender will burst forward with the long gun's barrel, smashing it straight into the assailant's face or throat. To execute the defense properly, you must extend the long gun at the correct time and with considerable accuracy to damage the assailant before his overhead attacking arm comes forward. This defense uses a straight thrust to the assailant's solar plexus, throat, or face. It relies heavily on timing and is difficult if you are using a bull-pup or short SMG-designed weapon.

After thwarting the initial attack, continue with counterattacks, including additional long-gun combatives and a straight kick to the groin or side kick to the knee. You may move to the assailant's knife-arm side, immediately slashing at his knife arm to break it, or at least make him drop the weapon. If the assailant steps back, you may also go to the other side to stay away from the knife arm. The follow-up, as with all defenses, is dependent on how the assailant is affected by your initial combative.

Low Straight-Stab Preemptive Thrust

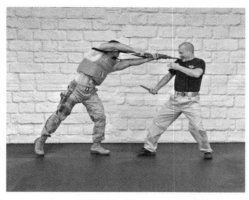

Thrust the muzzle straight into the assailant's face or throat. Continue with retzev combatives to disable the assailant, including smashing his knife-wielding arm to force him to drop the weapon. Of course, if the long gun is inoperable, render it operable or use a secondary weapon to shoot the adversary (as necessary and justified).

Low Straight-Stab Sidestep Defense

As with earlier straight-stab defenses, use a simultaneous sidestep and parry combined with a straight-thrust counterattack.

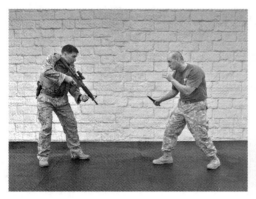 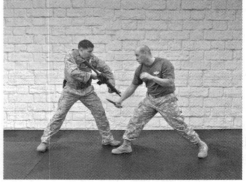

Recognize the assailant's grip of the edged weapon and, therefore, how it might be employed. From the low ready rifle position, raise the long gun and close on the assailant by sidestepping forward diagonally. Rotate the long gun down, angling it to use its length (topside) to intercept his straight stab. From the high ready rifle position this defense would be more time consuming, as you must lower the weapon; however, it is easily done, provided your timing and distance are adequate.

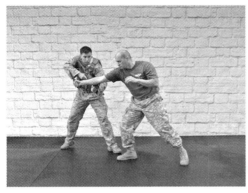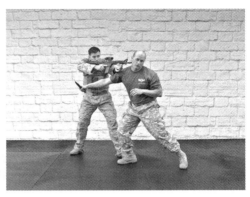

Smash the knife arm and allow it to slide along the barrel while you keep moving forward to the assailant's deadside. After deflecting his strike, immediately thrust the muzzle into the assailant's head or face.

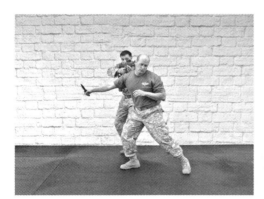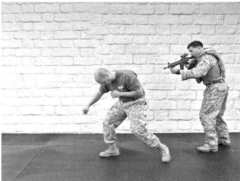

Keep moving to the assailant's deadside. Natural follow-on strikes include horizontal or uppercut butt strikes, provided a sling will allow these combatives. Continue with additional retzev combatives as necessary, or create distance, allowing you to render the long gun operable or deploy a secondary weapon.

Submachine Gun Sidestep Defense against a Straight Stab

An inoperable submachine gun may also be used effectively against a low straight stab by simultaneously sidestepping forward diagonally and parrying the weapon. Transition immediately into a counterattack such as a straight thrust to the assailant's head.

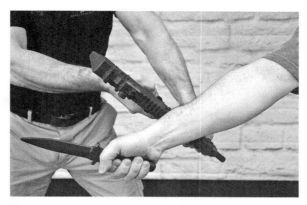

From the ready position, rotate the submachine gun down, angling the weapon to use its length (topside) to intercept his straight stab. Smash the knife arm and allow it to slide along the barrel while you keep moving forward to the assailant's deadside. After deflecting his incoming strike, immediately thrust the muzzle into the assailant's head or face. Keep moving to the assailant's deadside. Natural follow-on strikes include additional thrusts and slashes. Continue with additional retzev combatives as necessary or create distance to render the long gun operable or deploy a secondary weapon.

Straight Blocking Method (Less Preferred) against an Overhead Strike

It is possible to use a long gun to effectively deliver a parallel block against a low stab (and overhead stab). The previous low straight-stab defense accomplishes two key tactical goals: (1) parries the weapon and (2) takes the defender off the line of attack. Krav maga generally relies on combining a weapon deflection with a body defense. Note: this defense may not be possible if the long gun has a short sling.

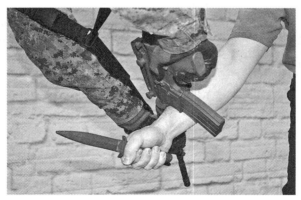

The defender uses the long gun—wielding it perpendicular to the stab—to stop the knife. Note, however, that the weapon is close to the body and the defender remains in front of the assailant with limited counterattack options. If the defender is wearing a Kevlar helmet, a head butt is a strong counterattack option.

Defending a Surprise Overhead Attack from the Rear

An obvious negative-five situation is an edged-weapon attack from the rear, or your six o'clock position. These defensive options require you to recognize his incoming attack with enough time to turn and intercept the assailant before the upraised knife hand comes down.

Rear Defensive Kick

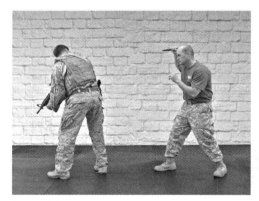 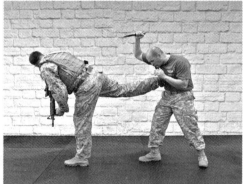

Recognizing the threat, stop the attack with a strong debilitating rear defensive kick, landing your heel against the assailant's groin or midsection. Immediately withdraw the leg and turn into a right outlet stance or your normal shooting platform.

Turn into Defensive Long-Gun Strike

If taken by surprise (negative five) from your twelve o'clock, you must obviously turn as quickly as possible to thwart the attack.

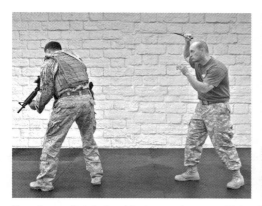 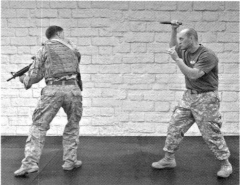

Turn immediately to sidestep and move off the line of his incoming attack.

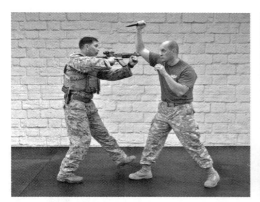 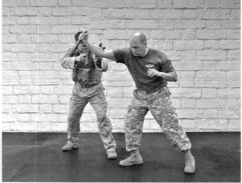

As you turn, sidestep the line of attack, bringing your long gun to bear in a cold-weapon capacity, and smash the assailant's arm.

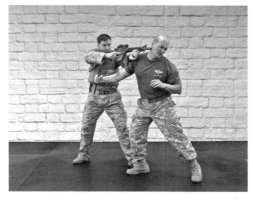

Shoot or use the weapon in a cold-weapon capacity to gain distance for a clear field of fire.

Another tactic that should be mentioned is if you are stabbed, a combat roll forward may be used to turn and face the assailant to use your long gun. The goal is never to get stabbed, but if you are stabbed once, move away to prevent multiple wounds.

Surprise Overhead Attack from the Rear (Not Depicted)

Similar to the underhand attack from the rear, deliver a straight midsection side kick to the assailant's torso or throat to stop the attack and pivot to shoot. You must immediately withdraw your leg and turn to press the attack with additional kicks or hand defenses if your long gun is not at the ready.

Long-Gun Preemptive Thrust Defense against a Forward Edged-Weapon Slash

Similar to the overhead and low straight stabs, a preemptive thrust may be used with correct timing.

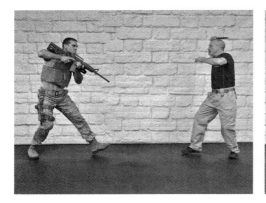 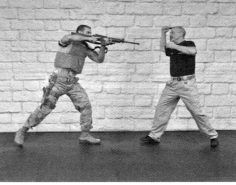

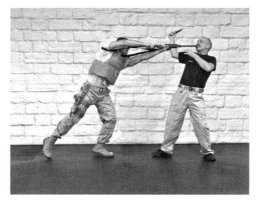

Recognize the assailant's grip of the edged weapon and, therefore, how it might be employed. Using timing to preempt the assailant's forward slash, lunge forward with the long gun's barrel.

Thrust the muzzle straight into the assailant's face or throat. Continue with additional retzev combatives as necessary or create distance to render the long gun operable or deploy a secondary weapon.

Long-Gun Defense against a Forward Slash

This defense using an inoperable long gun once again sidesteps off the line of attack to intercept his incoming knife arm followed immediately with a barrel slash to the assailant's throat or head and then additional combatives. The key once again is correct timing. Note that, once more by design, while the edged weapon presents a deadly threat, this defense is nearly identical to Inoperable Long Gun against a Hook Punch, along with the impact-weapon defenses against hook punches, which we saw earlier.

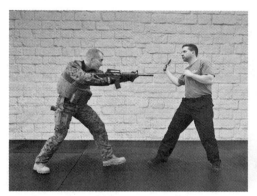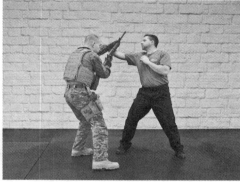

Recognize the assailant's grip of the edged weapon and, therefore, how it might be employed. From the ready position, as you recognize his incoming forward slash, sidestep away diagonally with your right foot, followed by your left foot. As you step, use the long gun to intercept his incoming arm.

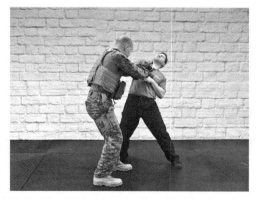

As you batter his extended arm, immediately transition to a slash to the assailant's head or neck. Natural follow-on strikes include horizontal or uppercut butt strikes (provided a sling will allow these combatives). Continue with additional retzev combatives as necessary or create distance to render the long gun operable or deploy a secondary weapon.

Long-Gun Defense against a Forward Slash, Variation

When the long gun is short barreled, has a broomstick type of foregrip, or a short sling (or all three), this variation of the forward slash defense inverts the long gun's muzzle down to intercept his forward slash.

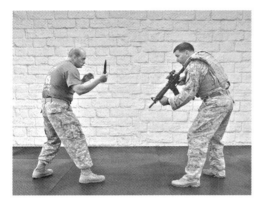
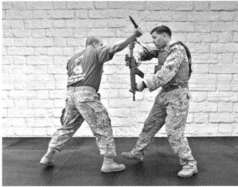

Recognize the assailant's grip of the edged weapon and, therefore, how it might be employed. From the low ready rifle position, extend your arms out to place the long gun as far away as possible from your frame to intercept his incoming slash. As you burst inside, use the length of the inverted long gun to intercept his incoming arm. From a high ready rifle position, this defense would be similar to Long-Gun Defense against a Forward Slash.

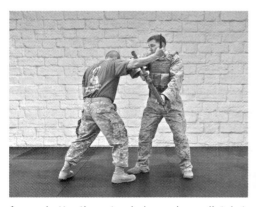
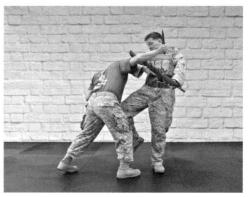

As you batter the extended arm, immediately transition to a knee or kick to the assailant's groin.

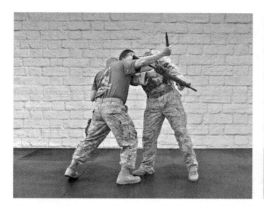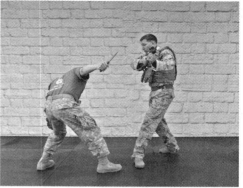

You may follow up with a head butt, especially if you are wearing a Kevlar helmet. Natural follow-on strikes include horizontal slashes or uppercut slashes with the barrel (provided a sling will allow these combatives). Continue with additional retzev combatives as necessary.

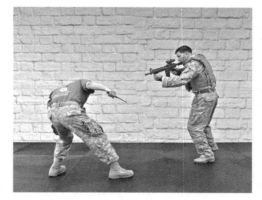

Create distance to render the long gun operable or deploy a secondary weapon.

Long Gun with a Short Barrel and Foregrip Forward Slash Defense, Machete Variation

Similar to defending against a forward knife slash, when defending against a forward machete slash—and if the long gun is short barreled, has a broomstick foregrip, or a short sling (or all three)—a variation of the forward slash defense inverts the long gun's muzzle down to intercept his forward slash. Your timing must be exceptionally good given the machete blade's length and consequent reach.

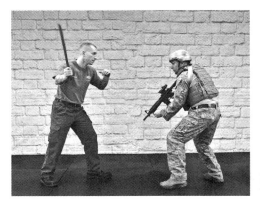 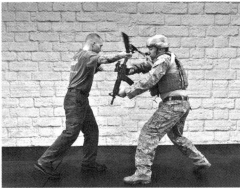

From the low ready rifle position, extend your arms out to place the long gun as far away as possible from your frame to intercept his slash. As you burst, use the length of the long gun to intercept or slash his incoming arm. From a high ready rifle position, this defense would be similar to Long-Gun Defense against a Forward Slash.

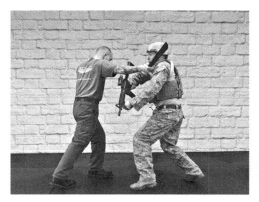 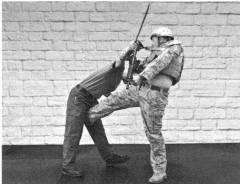

As you batter his extended arm, immediately transition to a longer-distance straight kick to his groin.

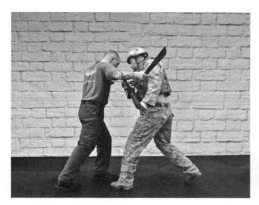 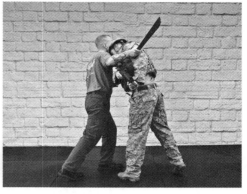

Instead of a straight kick, you may counterattack with a head butt, especially if you are wearing a Kevlar helmet. Natural follow-on strikes include horizontal slashes or uppercut types of slashes with the barrel (provided a sling will allow these combatives). Continue with additional retzev combatives as necessary. Create distance to render the long gun operable or deploy a secondary weapon.

Long-Gun Preemptive Thrust Defense against an Edged-Weapon Back Slash

Similar to the overhead attack, low straight stab, and forward slash, with correct timing a preemptive thrust with an inoperable long gun to the assailant's head may be used.

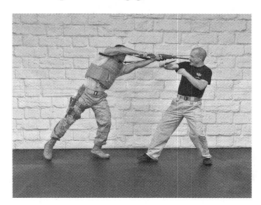

Using correct timing, preempt the assailant's back slash. Lunge forward with the long gun's barrel pointed at the assailant's head to thrust the muzzle straight into the assailant's face or throat. Continue with additional retzev combatives as necessary or create distance to render the long gun operable or deploy a secondary weapon.

Long Gun against a Straight Edged-Weapon Back Slash (Face to Face)

This defense uses the length of an inoperable long gun to intercept and jam the back slash arm, followed by an instantaneous straight-thrust counterattack.

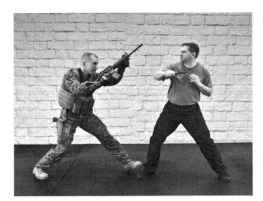 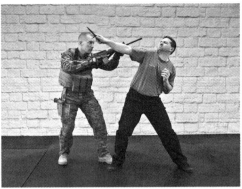

From a high ready rifle position, use correct timing to intercept the assailant's back slash by slashing your barrel into his arm. Then lunge forward to thrust with the long gun's barrel.

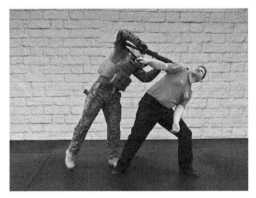

Immediately transition to a muzzle thrust straight into the assailant's face or neck. Continue with additional retzev combatives as necessary or create distance to render the long gun operable or deploy a secondary weapon.

Long Gun against a Long Gun (Cold-Weapon Capacity)

Krav maga's "rifle vs. rifle" (bayonet vs. bayonet) defenses are similar to those of many other military systems—great minds think alike. Developed as a military discipline, this training is an integral part of the krav maga curriculum. One difference is that professional krav maga incorporates low-line kicks with parrying and the accompanying long-gun combatives. As always, correct timing is the key in sidestepping off the line and parrying with a counterthrust, followed by additional combatives.

Rifle (Bayonet) against Rifle (Bayonet) Straight-Thrust Parry

As noted previously, krav maga has adapted to suit any type of long gun or submachine gun as required in a cold-weapon capacity, including "rifle versus rifle."

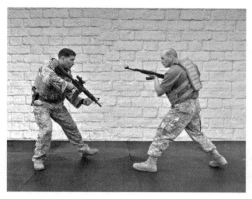 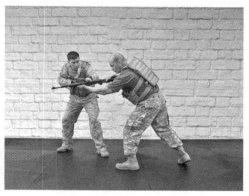

From the low ready rifle position, to defend against a straight-line thrust, move off the line with a diagonal forward sidestep while parrying his incoming thrust at a 30- to 45-degree angle, depending on the depth of your sidestep.

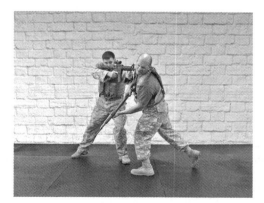

Transition immediately from the parry to a counterthrust. Redirect his parry and use the momentum to thrust your muzzle into his throat or face, followed by additional rifle and lower-body combatives. Continue with additional retzev combatives as necessary or create distance to render the long gun operable.

Rifle (Bayonet) against Rifle (Bayonet) Diagonal Slash Defense

To defend against this attack, use a diagonal forward sidestep to the liveside while bringing your own weapon up to intercept or counterslash the opponent's incoming slashing arm.

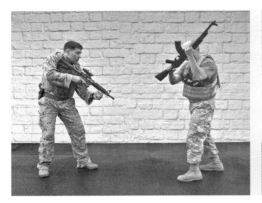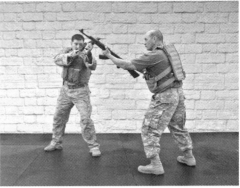

To defend against a diagonal slash, from the low ready rifle position, sidestep off the line while intercepting and parrying his incoming slash. In essence, counterslash to intercept his incoming strike. Another option is to invert the rifle so the length of the top of the weapon intercepts the strike and then proceed with your own counterstrike.

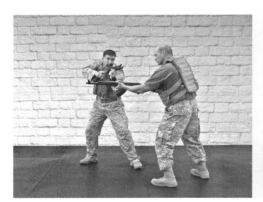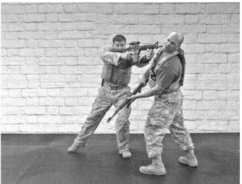

Transition immediately from the slash-parry to a counterthrust. Use the momentum of the parry to redirect the muzzle of your barrel into the assailant's throat or face, followed by additional rifle and lower-body combatives. Continue with additional retzev combatives as necessary or create distance to render the long gun operable.

Rifle (Bayonet) against Rifle (Bayonet) Horizontal Butt Strike Defense

To defend against this attack, you must burst directly into the opponent, placing your long gun's muzzle perpendicular to the ground to intercept his incoming strike. You may follow up with long-gun combatives or alternatively with a lower-body combative to transition to additional long-gun combatives.

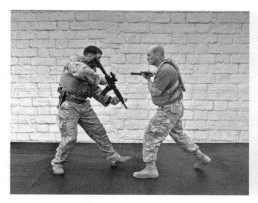 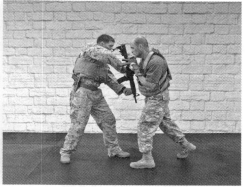

From the low ready rifle position, extend your arms and situate the long gun as far away as possible from your frame to intercept his incoming horizontal butt strike. As you burst inside, thrust the length of the long gun into his incoming weapon. Be sure to move both of your feet to transfer all of your body weight into intercepting his incoming strike.

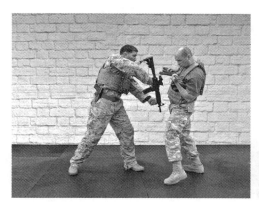 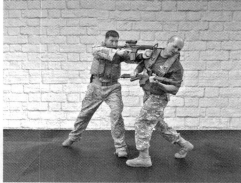

Jolt the assailant backward, using all of your body weight. As you create separation by driving the assailant back, thrust your weapon straight into his head, or you could deliver a groin strike with your forward leg. Natural follow-on strikes include horizontal slashes or uppercut slashes with the barrel (provided a sling will allow these combatives). Continue with additional retzev combatives as necessary. Create distance to render the long gun operable or deploy a secondary weapon.

Rifle against Rifle Magazine Strike Defense (Not Depicted)

This is almost identical to the defense we just discussed. Burst directly into the assailant, situating your long gun's muzzle perpendicular to the ground to intercept his strike. Follow up with long-gun combatives or alternatively use a lower-body combative to transition to additional long-gun combatives.

Rifle against Rifle Uppercut Butt Strike Defense

To defend against an uppercut butt strike (by design similar to the previous horizontal butt strike defense). As you intercept his incoming uppercut strike, use the momentum of the intercepting parry to redirect the muzzle of your barrel into the opponent's throat or face, followed by additional rifle- and lower-body combatives.

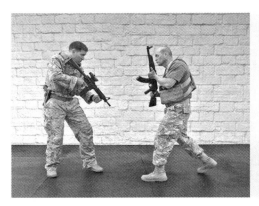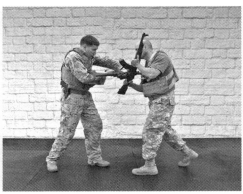

From the low ready rifle position, extend your arms out to situate the long gun as far away as possible from your frame when intercepting his uppercut butt strike. As you burst inside, thrust the length of the long gun into his incoming uppercut strike, or you could deliver a groin strike with your forward leg. Be sure to move both of your feet to transfer all of your body weight into intercepting his strike.

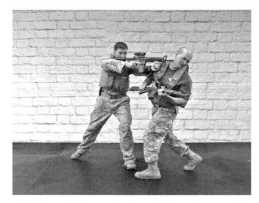

Jolt the assailant backward using all of your body weight and momentum. As you create separation by driving the assailant back, thrust your weapon straight into his head. Natural follow-on strikes include horizontal slashes or uppercut slashes with the barrel (provided a sling will allow these combatives). Continue with additional retzev combatives as necessary. Create distance to render the long gun operable or deploy a secondary weapon.

CHAPTER 6

Defending Edged Weapons: Open Handed and When Your Handgun Is Inoperable

Defense with an Empty or Malfunctioning Pistol against Edged-Weapon Attacks

When defending against an edged-weapon attack and your handgun fails, krav maga automatically switches to the same open-handed defenses used against such an attack. The difference, of course, is that you have a formidable short-length impact weapon. The defenses remain essentially the same. The difference is that the defender starts out expecting to use a hot weapon and has to transition automatically to a cold-weapon defense as the assailant makes his assault.

We will show a few examples of the most common attacks and how the handgun is incorporated into the respective defenses. For complete coverage, please refer to *Krav Maga Weapon Defenses* (YMAA, 2012), chapters 3 and 4. For those defenses not depicted in this book, simply substitute the handgun strikes for punches depicted in those chapters.

Overhead Edged-Weapon Attacks

Handgun Inoperable or Out of Ammunition: Straight Kick against an Overhead Attack

One of the most typical edged-weapon attacks is an overhand attack targeting the defender's neck. This technique follows the Tueller Rule that the average running assailant can cover twenty-one feet in approximately 1.5 seconds. If your handgun malfunctions, a strong kick to the groin in combination with a body defense and followed immediately with handgun cold combatives may be the best solution. Keep in mind that a kick to the groin will generally lurch the upper body forward while stopping the body's progress at the hips. A kick to the torso will jolt the body backward.

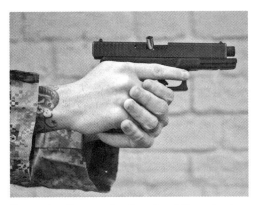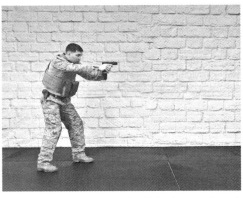

Recognize the assailant's grip of the edged weapon and, therefore, how it might be employed. Most important, after realizing your handgun is inoperable and as he closes on you, step off the line of attack to prevent the edged weapon from being plunged into you.

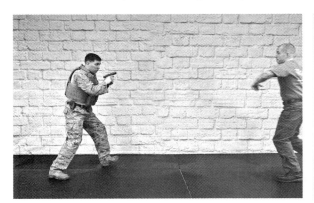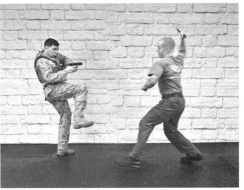

Using correct timing, step off the line and pivot your left foot 90 degrees (opening up the base leg), allowing the right hip and your whole body maximum follow-through. Stepping out into the pivot also allows for glicha, Hebrew for a sliding step, to drive the kick through the adversary with your body weight, generating optimum reach and power.

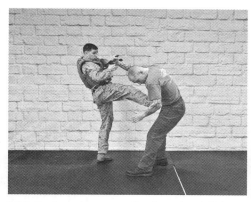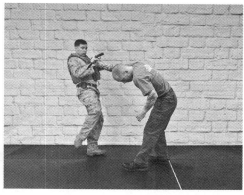

With the base leg correctly pivoted, a full-force kick to the groin or midsection will jolt the assailant's body, bringing the elbow of his edged-weapon arm either back to his torso or down and away from his torso. True to krav maga's philosophy of harnessing and honing the body's natural movements, the kicking leg will naturally retract on making contact. This is a crucial benefit because immediately retracting the leg will let you avoid being stabbed.

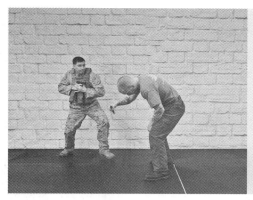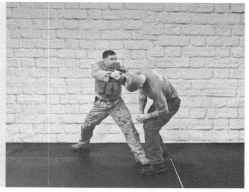

Press the counterattack by using the handgun to strike the assailant in the head or immediately create distance to render the handgun operable with a clear field of fire.

If the assailant jumps, use a straight defensive kick to his midsection or chest to drive him back. Follow up with another immediate left kick to his groin. Subsequent defenses (covered shortly) may be needed, depending on the situation.

Handgun Thrust against an Overhead Edged Weapon (Face to Face)

This defense uses a straight thrust to the assailant's throat or face while simultaneously stepping off the line. Notwithstanding this defense's effectiveness, it is risky. The defense relies heavily on timing and stepping off the line of attack just as the weapon is poised to strike or begins to arc downward. To be sure, this can be difficult if you are using a short-barreled handgun. To execute the defense properly, you must extend the handgun barrel at the correct time with full extension and considerable accuracy to damage the assailant before his overhead attacking arm comes forward. After thwarting the initial attack, continue with counterattacks.

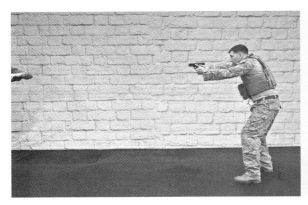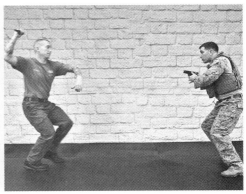

Recognize the assailant's grip of the edged weapon and, therefore, how it might be employed. Step off the line of attack with your arms coiled and your handgun prepared to thrust forward. Note: if you step too soon, the assailant can adjust his angle to put you squarely back in the line of attack.

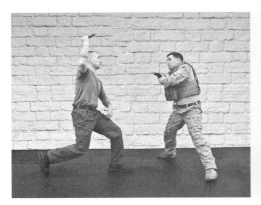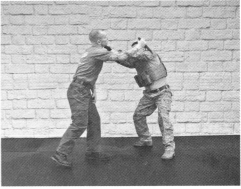

Using full extension, drive the barrel of your weapon into the adversary's face before he can swing down with his weapon.

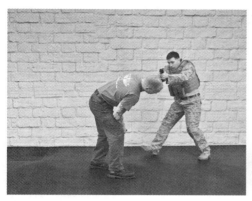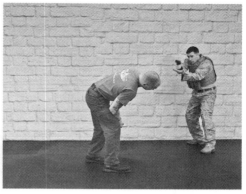

You may continue your counterattack with kicks or immediately create distance (as depicted) to place the handgun back into battery with a clear field of fire. If the assailant folds back as a result of your strike(s), you may also go to the other side to stay away from his knife arm. The follow up, as with all defenses, is dependent on how the assailant is affected by your initial combative.

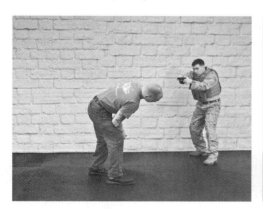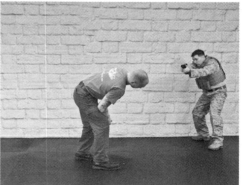

Create distance, tap the magazine, rack a new round, and assume a proper firing platform.

Handgun Inoperable Defense against an Overhead Stab (Face to Face)

Recall that krav maga's defenses must work for everyone and do not rely on strength. When confronting larger, stronger assailants, if you do not step off the line of attack, their superior body mass and strength could overcome your arm parry, even if you throw your body weight behind it. If you simply "burst" into the assailant, there is considerable risk you will be stabbed or slashed. Stepping out takes you off the line of attack and will work against an overhead long edged-weapon or a machete stab. When using a strong parry, you may find that your hand curves slightly upward. It is important to strive to deflect the punching arm as close as possible to the assailant's wrist and maintain contact with the assailant's arm after the initial parry. Parry or sidestep and counterattack, delivering a strong blow to the head.

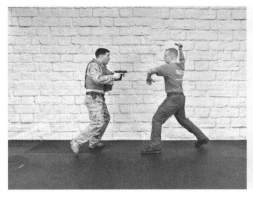 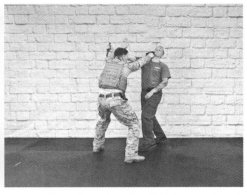

Recognize the assailant's grip of the edged weapon and, therefore, how it might be employed. Most importantly, after realizing your handgun is inoperable, step off the line of attack to prevent the edged weapon from being plunged into you. Although it is always better to step off the line of attack when you can, it is possible to step directly into the attacking arm as well. In other words, you may burst directly forward (not slightly to the side and forward) to intercept his arm while simultaneously smashing him in the face with your cold weapon. In either case, as you step, extend your nearside arm, chopping it into the assailant's incoming arm. As you step and chop, drive the muzzle of your handgun into the assailant's face or throat.

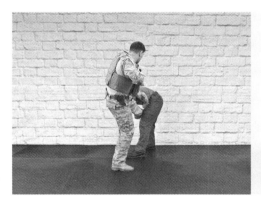 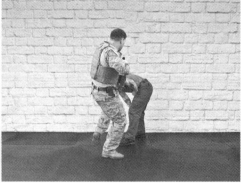

Continue your counterattack with kicks or immediately create distance (as depicted) to place the handgun back into battery with a clear field of fire.

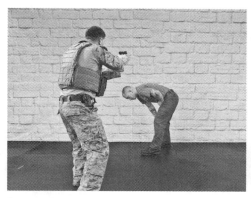 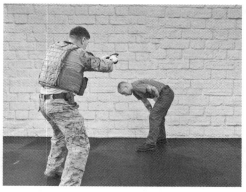

Create distance, tap the magazine, and rack a new round.

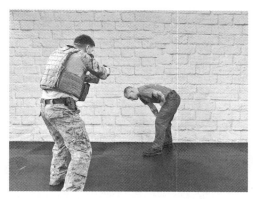

Assume a proper firing platform.

Holstered Weapon: Defending an Overhead Hook, Slash, or Edged-Weapon Attack with Handgun Deployment

This variation once again thwarts one of the most typical edged-weapon attacks: an overhead stab. Again by design, the same defense may also be used against a hook stab or horizontal slash when you are close and not in kicking range. This defense primarily relies on our instinct to parry and move away from a blow or, in this case, a hook punch. Notably, however, this defense will also work against an overhead edged-weapon attack, hook stab, or long slash. This law enforcement, professional security, or military-specific option incorporates the parry or sidestep and simultaneous counterattack to then immediately draw, aim, and shoot the assailant (provided the defender is wearing his sidearm on his right hip).

Understand clearly that parrying and simultaneously drawing the weapon is not an optimum tactic because the assailant is coming at you with full speed and force, more than likely with repeated stabs too, and you have not yet stunned him. Instead, you are relying on your ability to deploy and use your weapon, which, unfortunately, has had fatal consequences for many police and security officers. (A different tactic must be used if you have a sidearm on your left hip because your left draw hand must block and deflect the knife arm.) You should continue to move away from the edged-weapon arm. In summary, this defense can be combined with an initial strike to momentarily stun the assailant, create distance, and then deploy a firearm.

You may also burst directly into the arm rather than stepping off the line, but this variation requires truly exceptional timing and sufficient strength and body mass to stop his incoming weapon arm. Recall that krav maga's defenses must work for everyone and do not rely on strength.

In this scenario, you are caught in the negative five with your firearm holstered. You have demanded that the threat show his concealed hand, but you do not know what he is concealing behind his back.

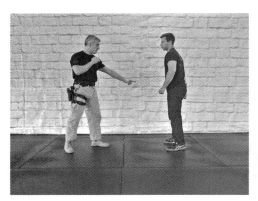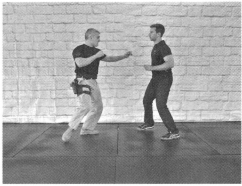

As soon as you recognize a forward arm motion, step off the line of attack to prevent the edged weapon from being plunged into you. As noted, although it is always better to step off the line of attack when you can, it is possible to step directly into the attacker to intercept his arm. Keep in mind that stepping away from the attack is just that. You are moving your upper body away or off the line from where the attacker intends you to be. If you simply burst into the attacker, you pit your strength against his. Krav maga makes a point of not pitting strength against strength. In either case, as you step, extend your nearside arm, chopping it into the assailant's incoming arm.

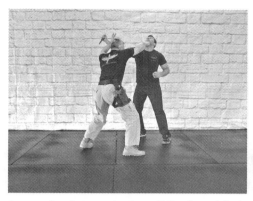 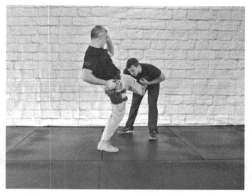

As you simultaneously step off the line while intercepting and blocking his incoming attack arm, strike the assailant in the face or throat. Continue your counterattack with a straight kick to the groin (preferably with your left leg, since the step will have loaded your weight onto your right leg).

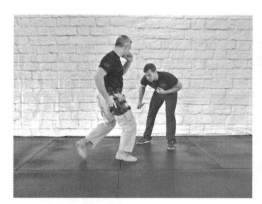 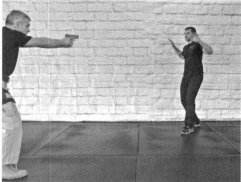

Immediately create distance as depicted to deploy your side arm with a clear field of fire.

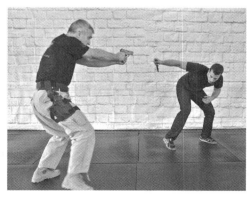

Fire as necessary if the assailant does not obey your commands or persists with his attack.

To reemphasize, on breaking contact, you can immediately deliver a swift, powerful left straight kick to the groin with a strong pivot on the base leg. This is a strong option because the assailant's arm will bounce off your deflecting arm and can be difficult to control. The sidestep places your right leg forward with your weight on it to take you off the line of attack. As your weight has now shifted, your left leg is positioned to deliver a debilitating left straight kick to the assailant's groin, allowing you to quickly disengage while continuing to break the angle (moving away from the edged weapon).

Holstered Weapon: Defending an Overhead, Hook, or Slash Edged-Weapon Attack with Immediate Handgun Deployment

While not an optimum defense, as discussed in the last section, this option may be instinctive for some armed personnel. To repeat a krav maga axiom: krav maga relies on a person's natural instincts. When facing a deadly threat, you are likely to instinctively reach for your sidearm. Krav maga recognizes this and builds on it. Again, this option's disadvantage is that you must be expertly trained to deploy your sidearm seamlessly while under the stress and pressure of a deadly force attack. An attempt to deploy a sidearm when there is no time—the very definition of a negative-five situation—has had fatal consequences for many police and security officers. (Note: if you have a sidearm on your left hip, you must use a different technique than the one depicted.)

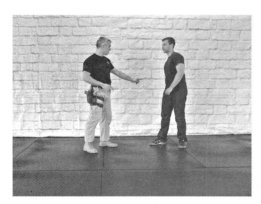 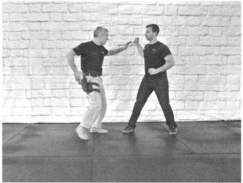

As soon as you recognize a forward arm motion, step off the line of attack to prevent the edged weapon from being plunged into you. As noted, although it is always better to step off the line of attack when you can, it is possible to step directly to the attacking arm as well. In other words, you burst forward using a direct movement to intercept his arm while simultaneously smashing him in the face with your cold weapon. In either case, as you step, extend your nearside arm, rotating and chopping it into the assailant's incoming arm.

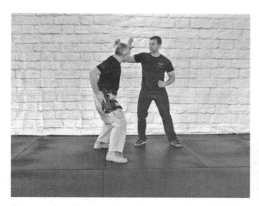 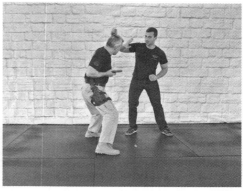

As you simultaneously step away from the incoming attack, deploy your sidearm and discharge it repeatedly as necessary, using your preferred point-shooting method or riding the weapon (discharging rounds into the body and the head). Be sure to keep your other arm up to defend against repeated stab attempts.

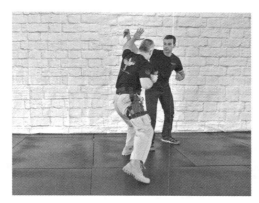

Despite the fact that the assailant has been shot repeatedly, there is a strong likelihood that he will continue his attempts to stab you. Keep your defensive arm up while you immediately create distance (as depicted) to continue point shooting until the threat is neutralized.

Note: in the unarmed version (when you do not have a handgun for cold-weapon combatives), the technique is exactly the same, except the defender delivers a punch to the assailant's face or throat. In this open-handed case, do not break contact with the assailant's knife arm. Close on the assailant with additional combatives for weapon removal, a control hold, or a cavalier to secure the weapon. (See *Krav Maga Weapon Defenses* [YMAA, 2012], chapter 1, for a review of control holds.) When caught by surprise, a fourth option is to step off the line of attack and deliver a raking combative to the eye ridge or a palm heel strike to the ear. At the same time, continue into a tai-sabaki movement away from the attack while deploying your sidearm.

Holstered Sidearm: Defending a Straight Stab Using an "L" Parry and Handgun Draw

This defense thwarts another typical edged-weapon attack, a straight stab to the body. You are caught in the negative five with your firearm holstered. You do not know what the threat is concealing behind his back (despite your demand that he show his hands).

To defend, your left arm leads the body to parry the straight trajectory of his arm as you sidestep. Your arm should be bent approximately 70 degrees to deflect-redirect the assailant's straight stab while making a subtle sidestep to the left. The parrying movement is no more than four to six inches and will lead the body's defensive movement—as with most krav maga defensive tactics.

This deflection-redirection is not an uncontrolled swipe or grab at the assailant's incoming arm—a common mistake when first learning the technique. The defensive arm makes use of the entire length of the forearm and up to the pinky to deflect any change in the height of the adversary's stab attempt. The movement rotates the wrist outward so your left thumb, kept alongside the hand with all the fingers pointing up, turns away from you as you make contact with the adversary's arm to redirect his incoming thrust.

After you parry and without breaking contact with the assailant's arm, which he will most likely retract, hook the assailant's arm by cupping your left hand, wrapping your left thumb around his forearm for control. Pin the arm against the assailant's torso while drawing and deploying your handgun. Keep in mind that the assailant may generate such momentum that you deflect and move deep into his deadside. Nevertheless, do not break contact with the edged-weapon arm, even if you cannot secure the arm and continue your retzev counterattacks. You are still safe, provided you are inside the arc of the edged-weapon attack (usually a backstab or back slash).

In short, the objective is to avoid being stabbed while placing you to the assailant's deadside with simultaneous deployment of your sidearm.

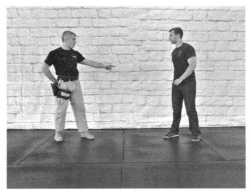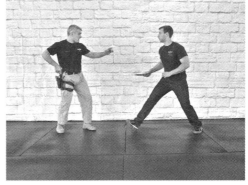

Recognize the assailant's grip of the edged weapon and, therefore, how it might be employed. Once more, as soon as you recognize a forward arm motion, step off the line to prevent the edged weapon from being plunged into you. Your left arm leads the body to parry the straight trajectory of his arm as you sidestep.

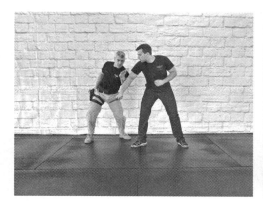 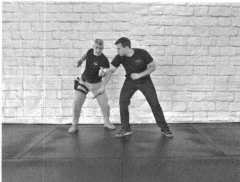

As you simultaneously sidestep and parry (note the deflecting arm's rotation), deploy your sidearm and use it as a cold weapon. Or discharge it using your preferred point-shooting method, "riding" or discharging the weapon into the body in an upward trajectory until a chin or headshot is achieved. Block the assailant's incoming attack arm and strike him in the face. Note: as an alternative to this technique, sidestep and deflect the attacker's weapon while counterattacking with open-hand combatives to the head. Keep moving to his deadside. Push him away as far as you can to gain time and distance to draw your firearm (not depicted).

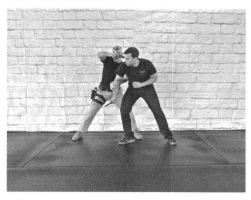

While creating distance, fire your weapon as necessary if the assailant does not obey your commands or persists with his attack.

The technique is the same for defending against a low straight stab; however, you should drop to the adversary's level by bending your knees. Beware of feints where the adversary initially motions low and then stabs high. Feints with a knife are very difficult to defend.

You must be prepared with the correct body positioning, and you must understand the most common feints—armed or unarmed.

Holstered Sidearm: Sidestep and Handgun Draw against an Underhand Stab

In this defense, the defender sees the edged weapon held in a low ready rifle position (similar to the previous straight-stab defense). This technique thwarts one of the most typical edged-weapon attacks: an underhand stab to the body. It varies slightly from the previous "L" block defense in two respects: (1) the blocking angle is the second movement of the "L" block (foregoing the slight arm chop or rotation), and (2) the defender administers a punch to the head before drawing. (Author's note: I felt it was important to depict both defensive options: first an immediate draw and then a strike and a draw.) Using either technique, your objective is to avoid being stabbed while simultaneously placing you to the assailant's deadside for deployment of your sidearm.

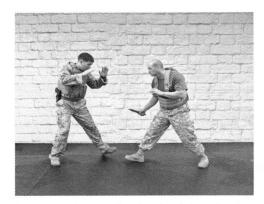 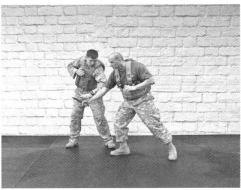

Recognize the assailant's grip of the edged weapon and, therefore, how it might be employed. Once more, as soon as you recognize a forward arm motion, sidestep forward diagonally. At the same time, use an angled forearm block to deflect-redirect the weapon. Also launch simultaneous punches to the assailant's head. Your left arm leads the body to block the low, upward straight trajectory of his arm as you sidestep. The angled parry creates a "V" with your arm over the top of the attacking arm while securing the assailant's wrist. The target for your parrying arm is just above the assailant's wrist, where one would normally wear a wristwatch.

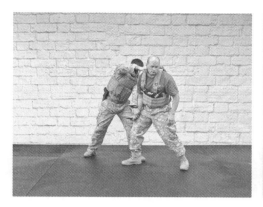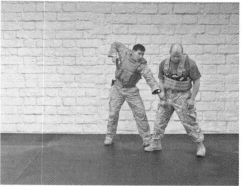

As you simultaneously sidestep and block, do not break contact with the weapon arm. Your counterstrikes should stun your assailant and allow you to press the handgun combatives counterattack. Note: as an alternative to this technique, sidestep and deflect the attacker's weapon while counterattacking with open-hand combatives to the head. Keep moving to his deadside. Push him away as far as you can to gain time and distance to draw your firearm (not depicted).

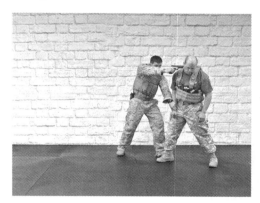

Deploy your sidearm and use it as necessary.

Defending a Forward Slash and Back Slash with an Out-of-Battery Handgun

An inside slash against the throat is another common attack. The following defense relies on a body defense and retreat to avoid the slash and an immediate counterattack as soon as the blade passes your throat during the assailant's forward slash. The goal is to pull your upper body back and, as the weapon moves past you, immediately burst into the assailant's arm to thrust your handgun into his head. Continue to move to the assailant's deadside and away as you deliver additional combatives and attempt to make your handgun operable once again.

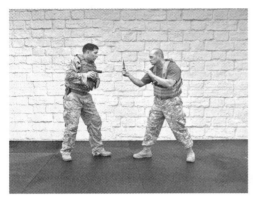 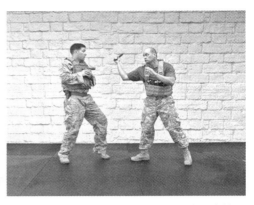

Recognize the assailant's grip of the edged weapon and, therefore, how it might be employed. Your inoperable handgun is at the close ready position. As soon as you see the forward arc of the knife, raise up on the ball of your front foot to help you move back and away from the knife's arc.

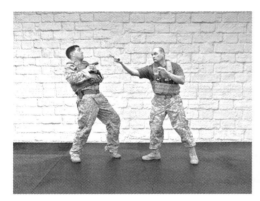 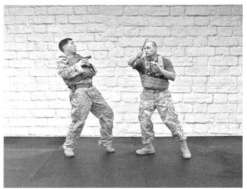

As the blade passes, immediately shift your weight back onto your front foot to burst into the assailant while preparing to thrust your handgun into his head. The "A" frame of your arms serves to defend against the back slash.

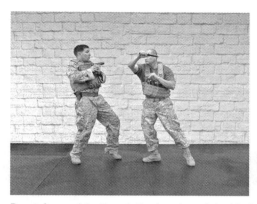
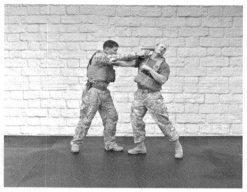

Burst forward to thrust the handgun into his head. Retreat and place the handgun back into battery. As an alternative you may also use your left arm to block the incoming slash while attacking the head with an open hand. (For an open-hand variation, see Two Assailants Armed with Edged Weapons, Variation 3, in chapter 7.)

Body Defense against an Inside Reverse-Grip Forward Slash and Reverse Stab with an Out-of-Battery Handgun

This defense is similar to the preceding forward slash defense. When a defender uses correct timing retreats to avoid the initial forward slash, a reverse back stab usually follows as the assailant continues to press his attack. Accordingly, retreat and then immediately burst back in with decisive handgun counterattacks to stop the attack.

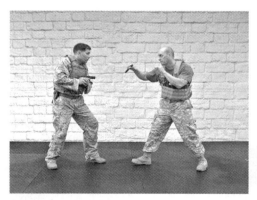
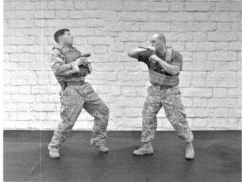

Recognize the assailant's grip of the edged weapon and determine how it might be employed. With your inoperable handgun at the close ready position, as soon as you see the forward arc of the knife, raise up on the ball of your front foot to facilitate your ability to move back and away from the knife's arc.

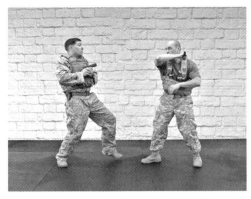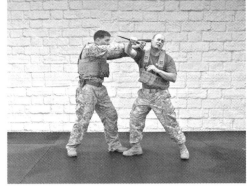

As the blade passes, immediately shift your weight back onto your front foot to burst into the assailant while preparing to thrust your handgun into his head. The "A" frame of your arms serves to defend against the back slash. Burst forward to thrust the handgun into his head. Continue with combatives or retreat and place the handgun back into battery. As an alternative you may also use your left arm to block the incoming reverse stab while attacking the head with an open hand. (For an open-hand variation, see *Krav Maga Weapon Defenses* [YMAA, 2012], pages 113–114.)

Note: this defense would be the same using a baton or even another edged weapon against a back slash, employing different counterattacks and weapon-disarming techniques.

Body Defense against a Back Slash and Follow-Up Forward Slash with an Inoperable Handgun

This defense is similar to the two previous defenses, except you retreat from the back slash and then close to intercept the forward slash. (See *Krav Maga Weapon Defenses* [YMAA, 2012], pages 116–117, for an additional comprehensive photo series depicting the open-handed version of this defense.)

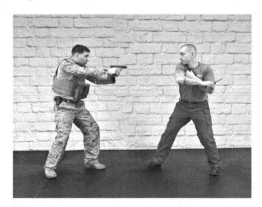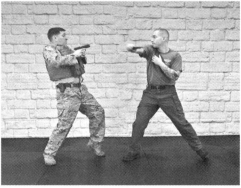

Recognize the assailant's grip of the edged weapon and, therefore, how it might be employed. Your inoperable handgun is at the close ready position. As soon as you recognize an incoming back slash, raise up on the ball of your front foot to help you move back and away from the knife's arc.

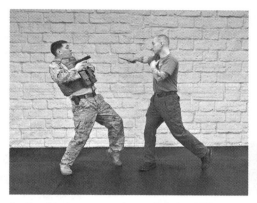 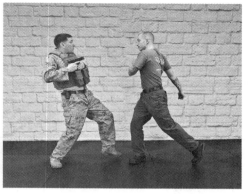

As the blade passes, immediately shift your weight back onto your front foot to burst into the assailant while preparing to thrust your handgun into his head. As you burst in while simultaneously stepping off the line, prepare your nearside arm to intercept the follow-up forward slash.

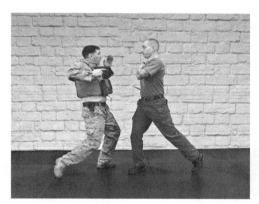 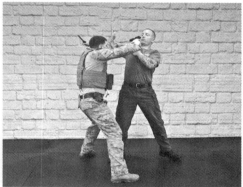

Burst forward to block the follow-up slash while thrusting the handgun into his head.

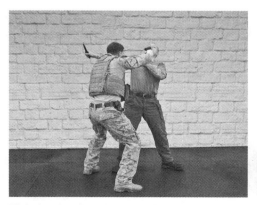 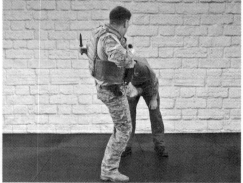

Kick the assailant in the groin and retreat to place your handgun back into battery.

Holstered Handgun: Defending against a Forward Slash

By design, this defense is similar to Handgun Inoperable Defense against an Overhead Stab (Face to Face). You are caught in the negative five with your firearm holstered. You do not know what the threat has concealed behind his back (despite your demand that he show his hands). As you recognize the incoming slash, your immediate step off the line is absolutely critical to defend against the forward slash. This is especially true when the assailant uses a short slash, keeping the elbow of his slashing arm close to his body. If you directly burst in, you will get lacerated.

As noted previously, it is always preferable to strike the assailant in the head to momentarily short-circuit his ability to continue attacking you. However, in this variation, we are focusing on an armed defender who naturally reaches for his sidearm. In other words, this tactic is based on the instinctive reaction that some defenders may take if they have not perfected the simultaneous defend-and-strike krav maga methodology.

As emphasized earlier, when defending an overhead attack, it is paramount to take a step away from the attack and then drive the assailant's arm back for control. Again, after stepping off the line of attack, driving the assailant's arm back serves two purposes: (1) it prevents the assailant from making further stabs and (2) it positions you to point shoot. Note: from extreme close range, you must use the quickest means to intercept or parry: an angled elbow gunt defense combined with a simultaneous handgun draw and point shoot.

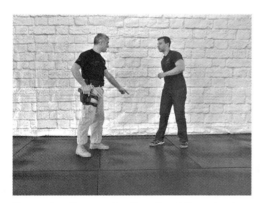 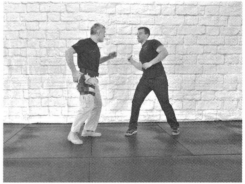

Recognize the assailant's grip of the edged weapon and, therefore, how it might be employed. As soon as you see the forward arm move, step off the line of attack to prevent the edged weapon from reaching you. As noted, although it is always better to step off the line of attack when you can, it is possible to step directly into blocking the attacker's arm as well. In either case, as you step, extend your nearside arm, chopping it into the assailant's incoming arm.

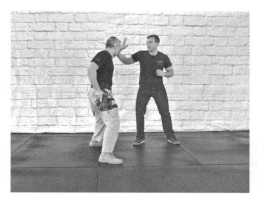
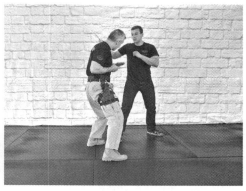

As you step, deploy your sidearm and discharge it, using your preferred point-shooting method, "riding" or discharging the weapon into the body in an upward trajectory until a chin or head-shot is achieved. Be sure to keep your defending arm up to counter his continued slash attempts.

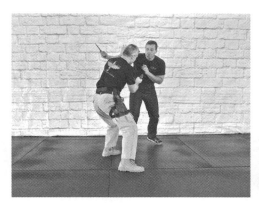
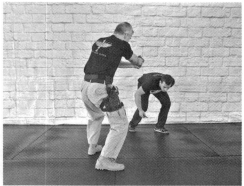

As you keep your defensive arm up, create distance (as depicted) to continue point shooting. Fire as necessary if the assailant does not obey your commands or persists with his attack.

Note: from extreme close range, you must use the quickest intercept or parry: an angled elbow gunt block defense (see *Krav Maga Weapon Defenses* [YMAA], pages 110–111). Combine this gunt with a simultaneous handgun draw and point shoot. There is a wide variety of these dangerous slash-and-stab attack options. If you cannot control the weapon with your initial defense, remember this: follow or defend against the most logical attack pattern or natural progression of the edged weapon after it is parried. As always, secure the edged weapon as soon as possible while initiating the most direct opportunistic counter-attacks.

Hostage Taker Holding a Knife to a Hostage's Throat

Neutralizing a Third Party Threatening with an Edged Weapon in a Hostage Situation

When there is no other choice—no "bullet to the head" option—but to attempt disarming a third party threatening a hostage with an edged weapon, you may wish to disarm the hostage taker from the rear, using a specific edged-weapon-removal technique combined with tai-sabaki. You must approach as silently as possible. Be aware that your approach could cast a shadow the hostage taker might see, or he might hear your steps. This takeaway requires great timing and precision. Against a right-handed hostage taker, your final step before attempting the disarming technique must be with your right foot to enable the tai-sabaki takeaway.

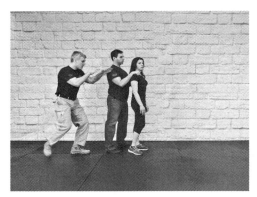 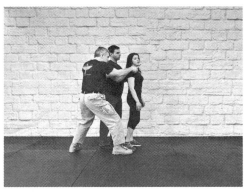

Step with your left foot positioned parallel to the hostage taker's legs. Secure his right arm with your left arm above his wrist while your right hand, using an underhand grip, secures the back of the hostage taker's hand using a knuckle-to-knuckle grip. Both of your hands must clamp down simultaneously on the hostage taker's right arm.

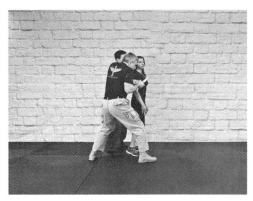 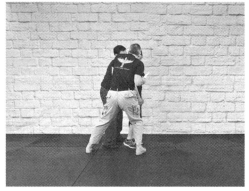

Immediately after clamping down, step forward with your right leg to execute Cavalier #1, forcefully taking down the hostage taker. Wrench the edged weapon back and away from the hostage's neck or throat, using the power of the cavalier and tai-sabaki movement. Do this with precision, since the blade must be diverted decisively away from the hostage's throat with dominant and secure control of the knife hand.

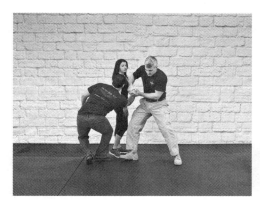 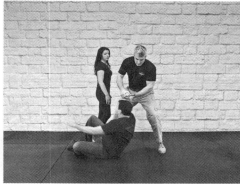

Follow through with Cavalier #1, keeping your elbows as close as possible to your body to best control the weapon, keeping it away from you and directed toward the assailant. Drive the assailant's pointer finger toward his same-side shoulder. Take a 180-degree rear tai-sabaki step with your left leg.

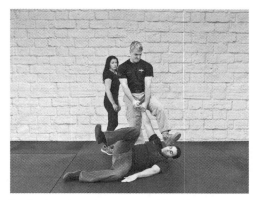

Kick the hostage taker in the head as necessary while disarming him by punching his wrist forward and down, allowing you to peel the weapon back and out of his grip.

CHAPTER 7
Multiple Assailants

The axiom that street violence is volatile and unpredictable could not hold truer than when facing multiple assailants. Facing multiple assailants, let alone multiple armed assailants, is an extremely dangerous proposition. Try to recognize the situation as soon as possible, such as if two people are walking toward you and suddenly fan out to your left and right. Running and escaping is your best solution.

If you cannot escape, there are two cardinal rules you must follow: (1) do not place yourself between two or more assailants and (2) do not end up on the ground. Tactically, to defend against multiple assailants, always use flanking maneuvers. In other words, if an assailant initiates to your left or right, engage him while keeping him in between you and any other assailants. If facing three or more assailants, even if you are attacked by the assailant in the middle, still move to one of your flanks. Never engage an assailant if the defense would put you in between two or more assailants. Techniques and tactics do not change, but you must modify your defenses to keep an opponent between you and any other assailants as long and as often as you can.

When defending against multiple assailants, Imi Lichtenfeld and Haim Gidon emphasize using optimum combatives to debilitate an opponent. Be it a kick, punch, elbow strike, knee strike, or eye gouge, every combative must count. The defender must maximize his power to debilitate, maim, or, if necessary, kill an opponent both brutally and efficiently in preparation for the onslaught of the next opponent. Of course, if you debilitate, maim, or kill an opponent quickly and decisively, his colleagues may think better of tangling with you; however, you may also increase their motivation to harm you. The bottom line, though, is that you should consider a multiple-assailant assault a threat to your life—period. Act accordingly.

One strategy is to target the "ringleader" to potentially sap an aggressive group's collective will to engage you. If you disable the leader, the others may think twice about pressing the assault.

You must keep your footing and balance to avoid falling or being dragged to the ground. If you are dragged to the ground, you must get up immediately. As the situation unfolds and necessity dictates, it may behoove you to put your back up against a solid object to prevent anyone from attacking you from the rear. This, however, hampers your mobility, so you should only do it as long as it is necessary.

It is paramount that you keep moving. Do not give the assailants a stationary target or any opportunity to coordinate their attack. The following photo series cannot depict a defender's constant movement, but you should assume the defender has kept moving and engaged the assailant(s) at the most advantageous moment.

The key for fighting multiple armed adversaries (and unarmed adversaries) is to neutralize one threat at a time, brutally and efficiently. To re-emphasize, you cannot get caught between two assailants. Engage one and disarm him immediately, optimally moving to his deadside. This is where proficiency in technique comes into sharp relief. You must neutralize and disarm the threat and immediately engage the other threat(s). Try always to position the first threat in between you and any other threat(s) to use him as an obstacle or barrier to shield you and buy time for you to gain the upper hand.

Note: all of the following scenarios assume you must defend open handed; you do not have access to your own weapon or a weapon of opportunity.

One Defender against Three Assailants (All Unarmed)

Do not let any of the assailants surround you or place you in the middle of them. Keep moving. You are their target and obviously a moving target is harder to hit than a stationary one.

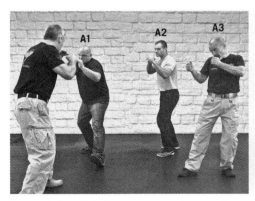 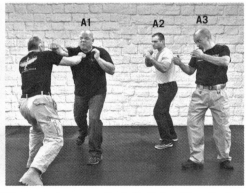

From a left outlet stance, engage the assailant (A1) closest to you on the left. Defend the straight punch using the parry and simultaneous counterpunch.

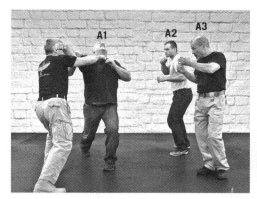 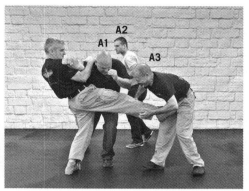

Counterpunch A1 while immediately preparing for the onslaught of the other two assailants (A2 and A3), noting that A2 is closer. As A2 closes, kick him in the groin with your nearside leg. Note: the defender is not in the middle as the A3 is still attempting to flank the defender.

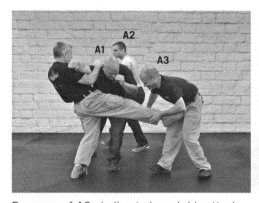 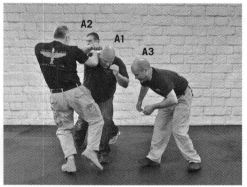

Be aware of A3 circling to launch his attack.

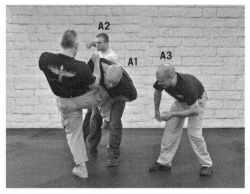 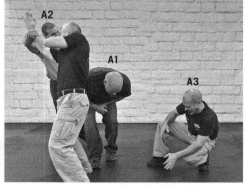

Continue to disable A1 with a straight groin kick while remaining aware of A3's movements. Use an inside "L" block and parry to defend A3's straight punch.

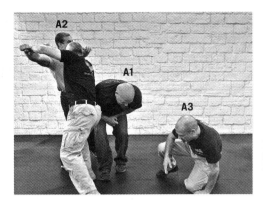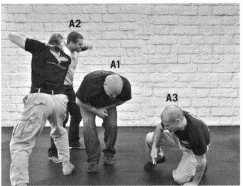

As you parry A3's incoming strike, immediately counterattack with a chop to his neck. Keep moving to the outside to create distance between the two felled attackers, A1 and A2, and keep yourself out of the middle.

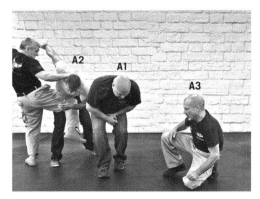

Keep moving away from the other assailants and knee A3 in the groin to further neutralize the threat. Make your escape.

Team Fighting against Multiple Assailants

If you and a companion must fight multiple assailants, the principles are the same as for an individual fighting multiple assailants—except you have a teammate to help in your counterassault. Defender 1 (D1) and defender 2 (D2) must coordinate their counterattacks. In other words, if D1 engages the outermost assailant (A1), D2 will loop behind D1 to help D1 attack the same outermost assailant, A1. For two defenders, when possible, the strategy should be for both to target the same opponent simultaneously; however, this may not always be possible. Alternatively, one defender may engage one opponent while the other defender moves to the first defender's rear to help the first defender or engage the next proximate opponent. In the depicted example, D1 and D2 will debilitate A1 and then move onto the next assailant (A2) to their flank. This will continue against a pack of assailants until the threat is no more or D1 and D2 can escape. D1 and D2 try not to get separated. For example, D1 does not fight multiple assailants while D2 fights another group of assailants unless absolutely necessary. Were this to happen, D1 and D2 should still make every attempt to link up, even midfight.

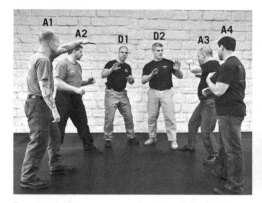 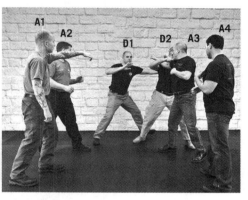

De-escalation or reasoning has failed. The group is intent on attacking. The most proximate assailant (A1) launches a straight punch at D1, who defends using the sliding parry and counterpunch.

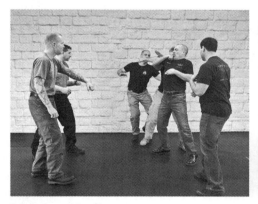 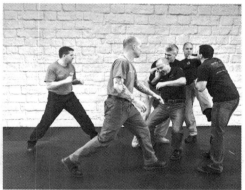

D2 follows D1 to immediately circle behind D1 and prepare for the next nearest assailant (A2).

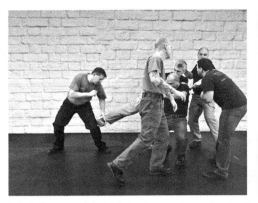 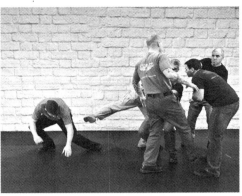

D1 delivers a side kick to the next proximate threat, the third assailant (A3), while D2 defends by kicking the assailant nearest to him.

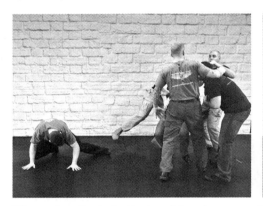 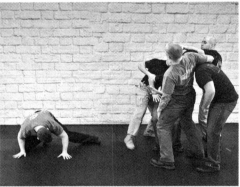

D2 punches the last attacker, A4 and prepares to disengage along with D1.

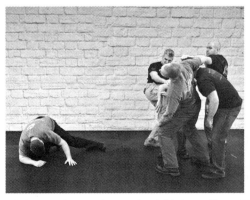 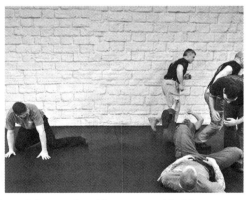

D1 further incapacitates the initial assailant, A1, and then makes his escape with D2.

Multiple Assailants Armed with Cold Weapons

When facing multiple armed assailants, you are veering closer to the negative-ten end of the scale. Defending against multiple assailants armed with cold weapons (impact and edged weapons) is, obviously, a precarious situation. To be sure, running and escaping is your best solution. Similar to defending against multiple unarmed assailants, if you cannot escape, there are two cardinal rules: (1) do not place yourself in between two or more assailants and (2) do not end up on the ground.

To defend against multiple assailants, always use flanking maneuvers. In other words, if an assailant initiates to your left or right, engage him while keeping him in between you and any other assailants. The general strategy is always to move to the deadside when possible, immediately debilitate the assailant, and remove the weapon to use against the second opponent as the situation dictates (see examples of previous techniques).

Both Assailants Armed with Impact Weapons

Begin in your left outlet stance. When contending against two assailants armed with impact weapons, follow the general krav maga strategy of engaging the most proximate threat.

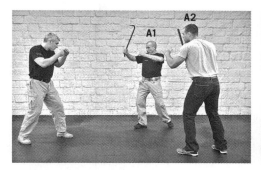 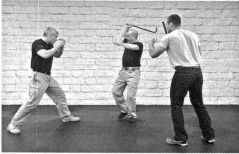

Initiate the defense by moving toward the closest assailant (A1).

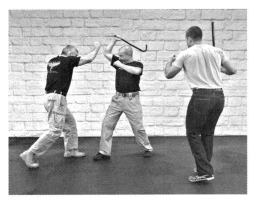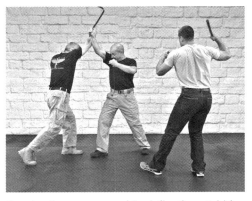

To defend against the overhead impact-weapon threat, align your nearside deflecting-stabbing hand with a forward body lean, burying your chin into your shoulder. Step toward A1 with the nearside leg and deflect with your nearside arm.

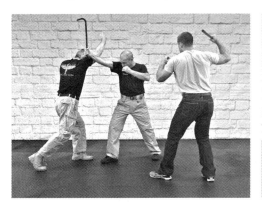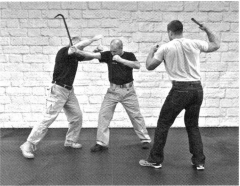

As the impact weapon glides harmlessly overhead off your shoulder and glances off your back, take a forward step with your rear leg without breaking your deflecting-stabbing arm's contact with A1's arm.

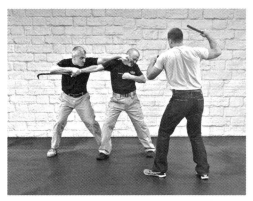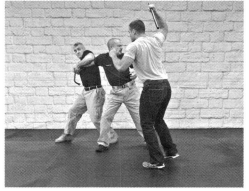

Turn your deflecting-stabbing arm's palm in and slide it down A1's arm, maintaining contact until you reach the assailant's wrist to secure it against his body while counterattacking with a straight punch to his head. To remove the impact weapon, the best option is to use a 180-degree step (tai-sabaki) with your right foot to break the impact weapon away from A1's hand without taking your eyes off him.

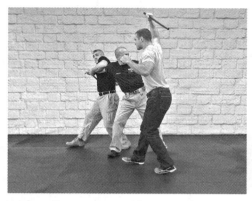 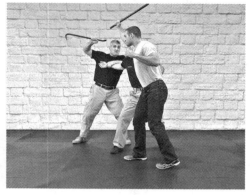

Remove the weapon and intercept the second assailant's (A2) overhead impact-weapon strike.

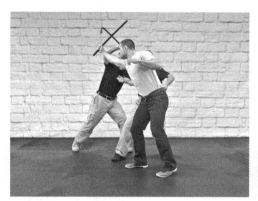 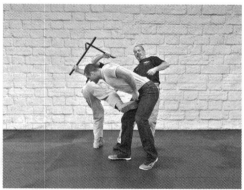

As you intercept A2's overhead strike, deliver a roundhouse kick, preferably with the ball of your foot to his groin.

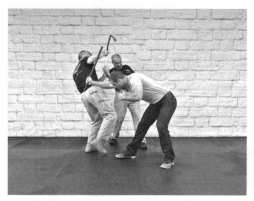 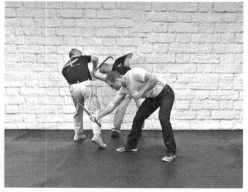

Continue to use the confiscated impact weapon as necessary to incapacitate or warn away any additional threat(s).

One Assailant Armed with an Impact Weapon and Another Assailant Armed with an Edged Weapon

In this scenario, disarming the assailant with the impact weapon may be preferable provided he is closer or equidistant to you than the edged-weapon threat. By using the preferred krav maga impact-weapon disarming technique, you can then use the impact weapon against the edged-weapon threat as covered previously in chapter 4.

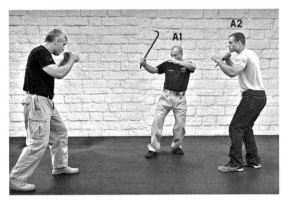
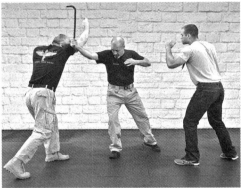

Recognize the grip of the closest assailant (A1) with the edged weapon and, therefore, how it might be employed. Initiate the defense by moving toward A1. To defend against the overhead impact-weapon threat, align your nearside deflecting-stabbing hand with a forward body lean, burying your chin into your shoulder. Step toward A1 with the nearside leg and deflect with your nearside arm. As the impact weapon glides harmlessly overhead off your shoulder and glances off your back, take a forward step with your rear leg without breaking your deflecting-stabbing arm's contact with A1's arm.

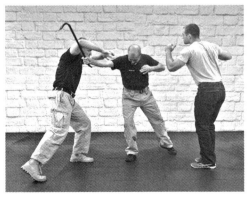
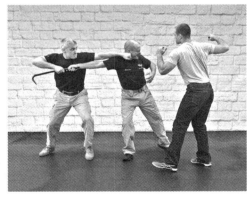

Turn in the palm of your deflecting-stabbing arm and slide it down A1's arm, maintaining contact until you reach the weapon. Secure A1's wrist to lock the weapon against your body while counterattacking with a straight punch to his head.

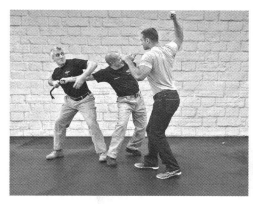 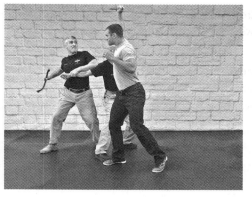

To remove the impact weapon, take an abbreviated 180-degree step (tai-sabaki) with your right foot to break the impact weapon away from his hand without taking your eyes off the second assailant (A2).

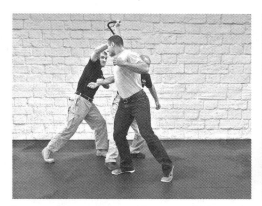 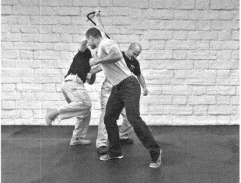

Remove the weapon and intercept A2's overhead edged-weapon stab attempt.

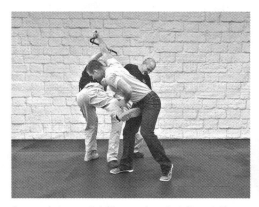 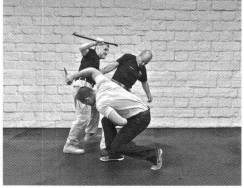

As you intercept A2's overhead strike, deliver a roundhouse kick, preferably with the ball of your foot, to A2's groin.

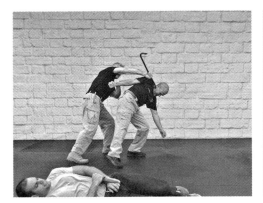
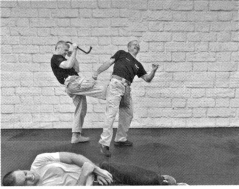

Continue to use the confiscated impact weapon as necessary and other combatives such as a kick to the groin to reduce the threat.

One Assailant Armed with an Impact Weapon and Another Assailant Armed with an Edged Weapon, Variation 1

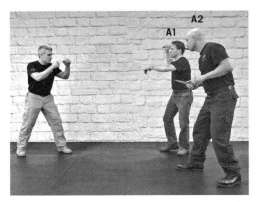
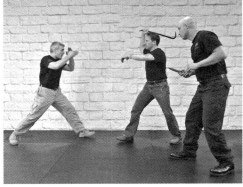

Recognize the grip of the nearest assailant (A1) with the edged weapon and, therefore, how it might be employed. Once again, initiate the defense by moving toward A1, the closest assailant. To defend against the overhead impact-weapon threat, align your nearside deflecting-stabbing hand with a forward body lean, burying your chin in your shoulder. Step toward A1 with your left front leg and deflect with your nearside right arm. As the impact weapon glides harmlessly overhead off your shoulder and glances off your back, take a forward step with your rear leg without breaking your deflecting-stabbing arm's contact with A1's arm.

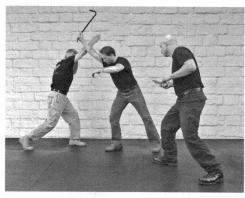 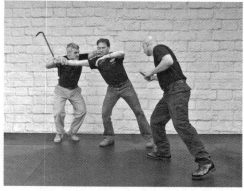

Turn in the palm of your deflecting-stabbing arm and slide it down A2's arm, maintaining contact until you reach the assailant's wrist.

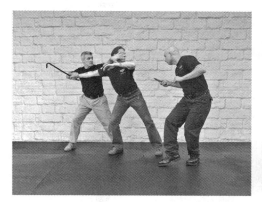 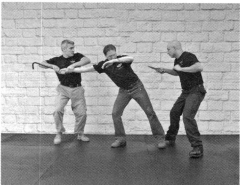

Secure A1's wrist against your body while counterattacking with a finger gouge deep into his nearest eye. After you gouge his eye, bring your left hand to secure his right wrist. Switch your right hand from his wrist to secure the weapon.

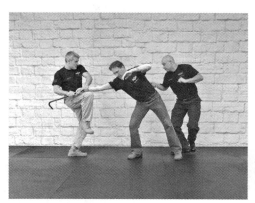 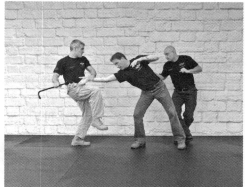

To remove the impact weapon, secure it with your right hand and use your right knee to smash his hand while simultaneously yanking the impact weapon down and out. Remove the weapon, keeping A1 in front of you while moving away from the second assailant (A2).

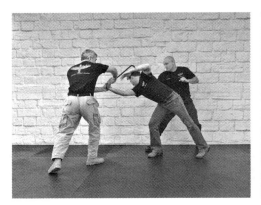
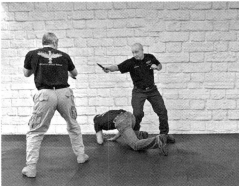

Secure the weapon and prepare it for use against A2.

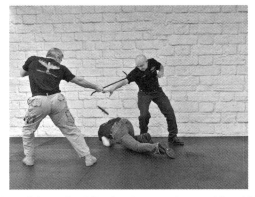

Sidestep the attempted straight stab while simultaneously smashing A2's arm. Continue to use the confiscated impact weapon as necessary.

One Assailant Armed with an Impact Weapon and Another Assailant Armed with an Edged Weapon, Variation 2

In this scenario, if the edged-weapon threat is closer or engages you first, perform the appropriate edged-weapon defense and confiscate the edged weapon. In a life-and-death scenario, the edged weapon may be used against the impact-weapon threat by simply modifying the impact-weapon defense.

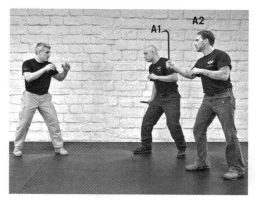 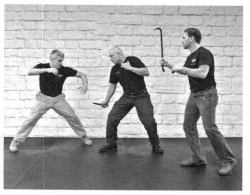

Recognize the grip of the edged weapon and how it might likely be employed. Once again, initiate the defense by moving toward the closest assailant (A1).

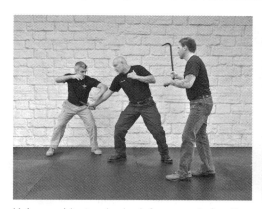 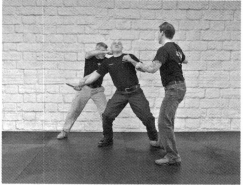

Using a sidestep body defense and simultaneous angled forearm block, deflect-redirect the weapon and launch a simultaneous punch to A1's head. The angled block creates a "V" with your arm overtop the attacking arm while securing A1's wrist. Your blocking arm targets just above A1's wrist where one would normally wear a wristwatch.

After the block and simultaneous counterpunches are delivered, without breaking contact secure the wrist while your counterattack arm now secures A1's hand for a Cavalier #1 weapon removal.

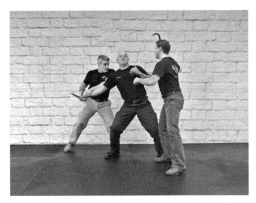 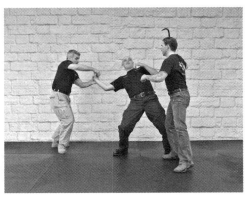

To remove the weapon from his grip using Cavalier #1, use the palm heel, placing your knuckles atop his knuckles to then punch his wrist toward him using your hips and upper body in concert. As you break the wrist's posture, dig your fingers into his palm, wrapping around the weapon's grip. Use your fingers to strip the weapon and pry it from his grip. Keep the first assailant in front of you while moving away from the second assailant.

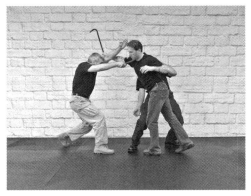

Secure the edged weapon and use the overhead stick defense (for a review see *Krav Maga Weapon Defenses* [YMAA, 2012], pages 27–29). Combine this with a weapon stab (instead of a punch) as necessary.

Two Assailants Armed with Edged Weapons

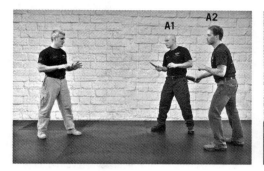 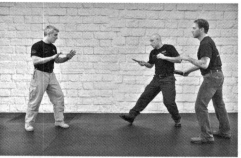

Recognize the underhand grips and how the weapons are most likely to be employed. Once again, initiate the defense by moving toward the closest assailant (A1).

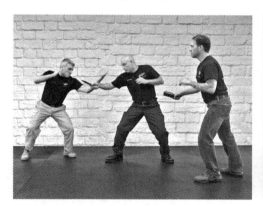 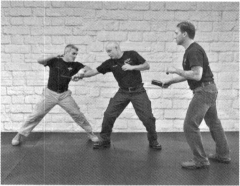

As soon as you recognize a forward arm motion, step off the line of attack and use the "L" block/parry to prevent the edged weapon from being plunged into you. Your left arm leads the body to parry the straight trajectory of A1's arm as you sidestep. As you deflect his incoming arm, instantaneously close on A1 to deliver a strong punch to his head. Use correct body mechanics (body weight delivery, hip pivot, and proper arm alignment) to deliver optimum power.

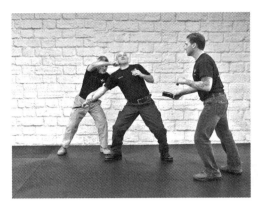 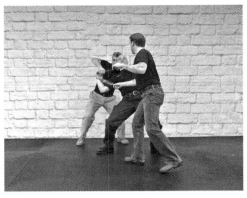

Strike A1 in the head and begin to move behind him, applying Cavalier #1 to remove the weapon from his grasp.

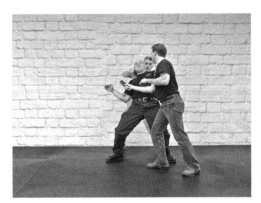 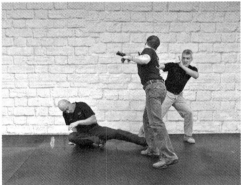

Remove the weapon with Cavalier #1. Use the weapon as necessary to disable A1. Keep A1 in front of you while moving away from A2. Slash A2's arm and move off the line as he attempts to stab you. Continue with retzev combatives as necessary.

Two Assailants Armed with Edged Weapons, Variation 1

Here, you must defend against two assailants both holding edged weapons with overhand grips.

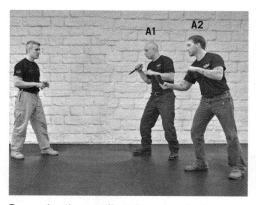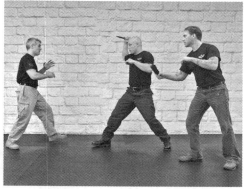

Recognize the assailants' overhand grips and how the weapons are most likely to be employed. Once again, initiate the defense by moving toward the closest assailant (A1). Moving to A1's deadside, take a left step while preparing an outside defense with your right arm. Your left arm is held in a supportive defensive position.

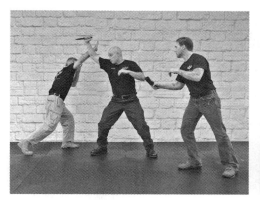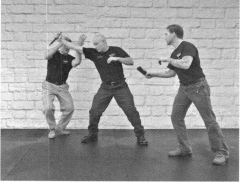

Forcefully deflect A1's incoming overhead strike with a strong outside rotation. As you deflect the stab attempt, sidestep and bring your left arm up to switch deflecting arms. With your left arm, continue to rotate the attacking arm away using a modified "L" block rotation.

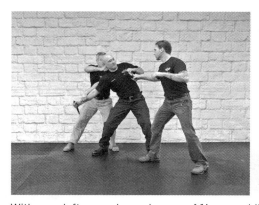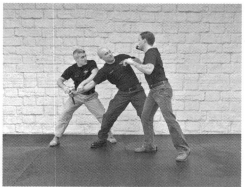

With your left arm, clamp down on A1's arm while forcefully punching him in the head. Remove the weapon using Cavalier #1 while keeping A1 in front of you and moving away from the second assailant (A2).

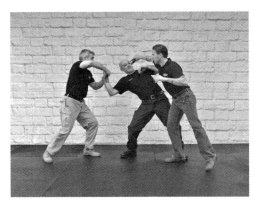 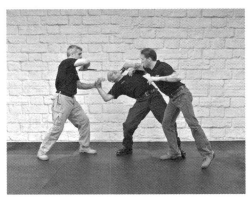

After removing the weapon, use it as necessary to disable A1.

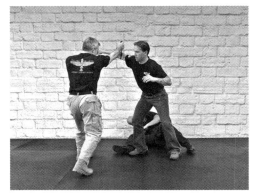

Use the edged weapon to defend against A2's hook-stab attack by intercepting and lacerating his arm. Continue to use the edged weapon if necessary.

Two Assailants Armed with Edged Weapons, Variation 2

You must defend against two assailants both holding edged weapons. One assailant (A1) has an underhand grip while the other assailant (A2) has an overhand grip.

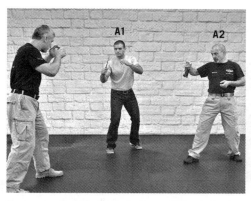
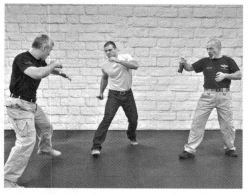

Recognize the kind of grip the assailants have and how each might employ his respective weapon. Once again, initiate the defense by moving toward the closest assailant (A1).

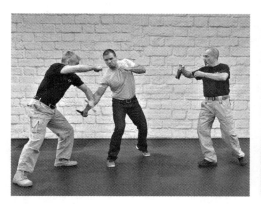
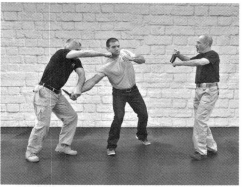

Using a sidestep body defense and simultaneous angled forearm block, deflect-redirect the weapon and launch a simultaneous punch to A1's head. The angled block creates a "V" with your arm overtop the attacking arm while securing A1's wrist. Your blocking arm targets just above A1's wrist where one would normally wear a wristwatch.

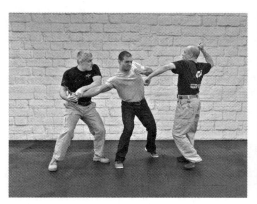
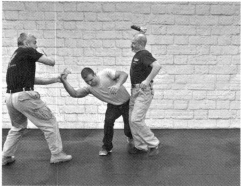

Once you deliver the block and simultaneous counterpunch—and without breaking contact— secure the wrist while your counterattack arm now secures the hand for a Cavalier #1 weapon removal. Keep A1 in front of you and move away from the second assailant (A2).

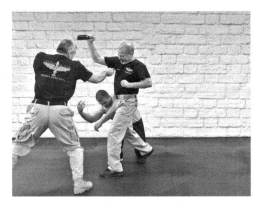

Use the weapon as necessary to defeat A2's incoming attack.

Two Assailants Armed with Edged Weapons, Variation 3

You must defend against two assailants both holding edged weapons. Both assailants have underhand grips.

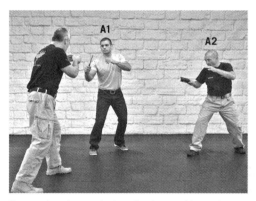 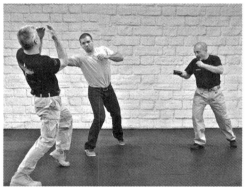

Recognize the underhand grips and how the assailants might use their weapons. In this scenario, you recognize that the more proximate assailant (A1) has his arm outstretched and holds the weapon as if to slash. A1 initiates a forward slash. Use a proper body defense by keeping your arms up (wrists facing you) and retreating on the ball of your front foot.

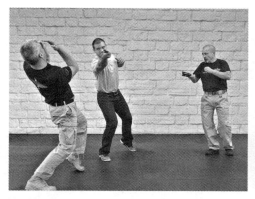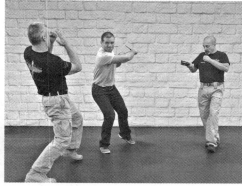

Having avoided the slash and as the knife arm passes you, prepare to burst in to jam A1's knife arm.

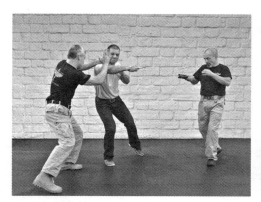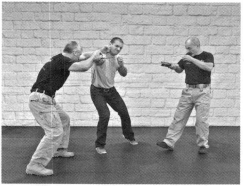

Keeping both hands up and positioned properly, close the distance and jam A1's knife arm with your left arm, driving your ulna through his arm while counterattacking with an over-the-top sliding punch.

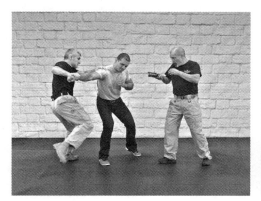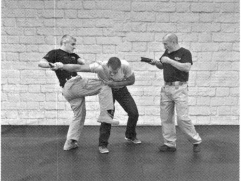

Deliver a strong straight knee to A1's midsection or thigh. Without breaking contact, secure the wrist while your counterattack arm now secures the hand for a Cavalier #1 weapon removal.

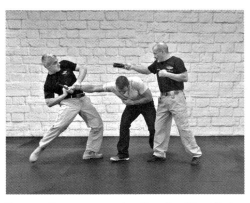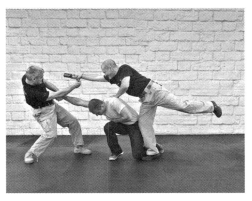

Remove the weapon using Cavalier #1 while keeping the first assailant in front of you and moving away from the second assailant (A2). Use the weapon as necessary to defeat A2's incoming straight stab attack.

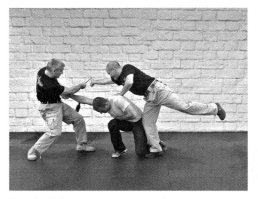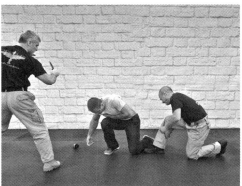

Decide if further counterattacks are necessary.

CHAPTER 8

Firearm Defenses

Krav Maga's Firearm Disarming Philosophy

The human brain slows down when processing several stimuli or engaged in thought processes. If you must disarm an assailant brandishing a handgun or long gun, the best time to act is when the assailant is distracted. Of course, in your attempt to disarm, the gunman now considers you a deadly threat and will fight as if his or her life is at stake. Firearms are ergonomically designed for the operator of the weapon—not someone trying to take the weapon away, especially if the operator has a two-handed vice grip on it. Therefore, whenever possible, it is advantageous to disarm a gunman from the rear or, at the very least, move deep to the gunman's deadside.

In nearly every instance, the firearm will discharge as you deflect-redirect it because of the assailant's reflexive trigger-press response. Make securing the weapon a priority and simultaneously neutralize your assailant with combatives to the throat, groin, eyes, and other secondary targets. As always, your krav maga must be decisive and brutally efficient while securing the firearm in the best possible way, reducing the chances of bystanders being shot.

Keep in mind that the assailant's immediate instinctive or flinch response will be to retract his gun and pull the trigger. Therefore, your strategy must also incorporate "time in motion." Time in motion is the movement pattern where the firearm (or any other type of weapon) is likely to end up as a result of your deflection-redirection and the assailant's reflexive response. Once again, it is evident why you must move deep to the deadside to keep yourself clear of the weapon's line of fire.

Once you have secured the handgun, if you have your own handgun, standard Israeli operating procedure is to revert to your own firearm. If you need to use the confiscated weapon, tap the magazine from the bottom (the insertion point into the grip) and then turn the handgun parallel to the ground to check the ejection port and rack a new round. After redirecting-deflecting and securing a semiautomatic handgun, rotate it 90 degrees, allowing gravity to help dispense a spent cartridge's case, which has likely jammed the weapon. Even if you do not tap and rack the handgun, which is likely to be inoperable, you should still consider it "live," or functional for cold weapon combatives.

Note: all of the following techniques assume the handgun is held in the assailant's right arm.

The Four Essential Components of Firearm Defenses

Disarming an assailant who is carrying a firearm is extremely difficult and dangerous. Be sure you have exhausted all compliance options and you have no choice but to attempt the disarming technique. If you decide there is no choice but to disarm an assailant, you must follow the four pillars of krav maga's firearm defenses:

1. Redirect-deflect the line of fire combined with a body defense.

2. Control the firearm whenever possible, moving deep to the deadside while stunning and neutralizing the assailant.

3. Understand "time in motion"—or what the gunman's reaction will be the instant you react.

4. Disarm the assailant and create distance, maintaining control of the firearm.

There are a myriad of angles and heights from which an assailant could deploy a firearm. The following disarming techniques cover the positions and angles of hand-guns commonly seen in a hostage or active-shooter scenario. They are presented as a blueprint against firearm threats.

Krav maga's philosophy is to adapt to a situation using core techniques and principles. If you find yourself in a situation not covered in this book, fall back on the above four pillars for firearm defenses and use common sense. You could find yourself defending against a handgun threat obscured by a magazine, newspaper, or cloth. The defensive principles remain the same; however, you must take into account that your grip and subsequent control on the handgun could slip. Therefore, your removal of the weapon must be modified to cope with the situation, such as removing it from underneath a garment (see *Krav Maga Weapon Defenses* [YMAA, 2012], pages 177–178). Also keep in mind that in your attempt to disarm, the assailant is likely to instinctively retract his arm. You must understand "time in motion"—both yours and his—or how a body instinctively reacts to a stimulus to properly time any disarming technique.

Note: for all firearm defenses, as you attempt to control the weapon, the gunman is likely to retract it and pull the trigger to discharge it.

For demonstration purposes of the book the handgun is often held without the trigger finger inserted. This is to prevent injury. Where necessary, the "assailant" has inserted his finger to show the specific removal technique. When practicing these techniques, determine with your partner if he or she will keep the trigger finger inserted.

Defense When the Handgun Is Visible in the Assailant's Front Waistband

An assailant could threaten you without deploying a handgun but by indicating or revealing its presence.

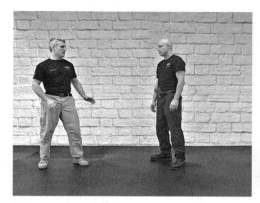 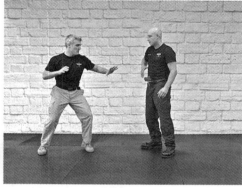

When you recognize the threat, react immediately by closing on the assailant to control his weapon hand and stun him.

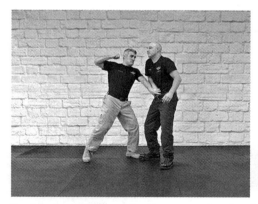 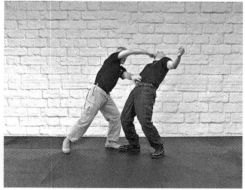

Decisively pin the assailant's weapon hand to his body. Control the handgun at the rear of the slide while delivering a forceful strike to the assailant's head. Note the importance of strong, effective combatives to disable the assailant prior to removing the weapon.

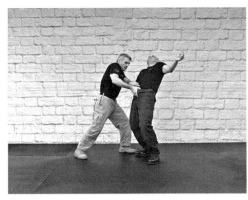 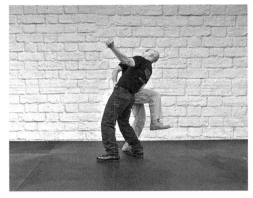

To secure the handgun, use your left arm to keep your weight pressed against the assailant's right wrist while clamping down with your right hand on the back of the assailant's hand on the grip. To remove the handgun, keep both of your hands securely attached to the assailant's right wrist and hand. Using a modified osoto-gari takedown, raise your right leg and step strongly between the assailant's legs.

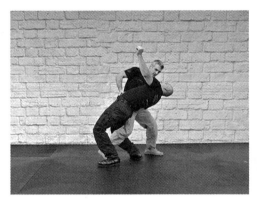 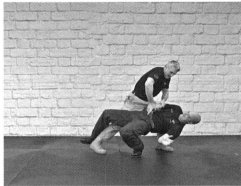

As you take down the assailant, be sure to keep your arms locked out to control the handgun.

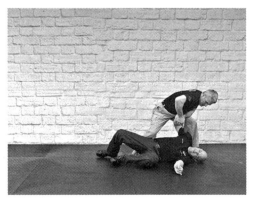 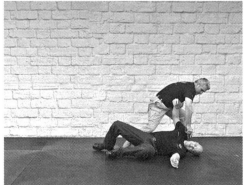

Remove the handgun and use it as necessary.

Note: the defense resembles Frontal Handgun Defense #1. See *Krav Maga Weapon Defenses* (YMAA, 2012), pages 158–163.

Defense When the Handgun Is in the Assailant's Rear Waistband

You could be threatened by an assailant reaching behind his back to retrieve a firearm (or other weapon) from his rear waistband. One defensive option is to kick the would-be assailant in the groin and then close on him. This allows you to close the distance with a knee strike to the groin or midsection while securing his reach arm with Control Hold #6, often called a *kimura* lock. You can also add a strong knee combative to take his level down.

The advantage of the combined knee combative and control hold is that you debilitate the assailant while maintaining control over his weapon arm. To finish the hold and maintain control of the weapon, you need to transition from controlling his forearm to controlling his wrist. Last, you turn the opponent on his side to prevent him from using his free arm to retrieve the weapon.

This technique sets up a prone variation of Control Hold #6. In this variation, you secure his arm while clamping down on his shoulder. You then release the closed guard momentarily to turn on your side and gain maximum positional control by reclosing the guard. You may also swing your underneath leg on top of him to avoid being pinned, using both legs to control him from the top.

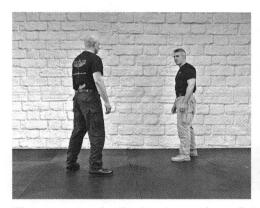 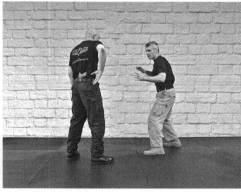

When you recognize the threat, react immediately with a diagonal left step to close on him and control his weapon arm and knee him in the groin or thigh (if use-of-force is a consideration).

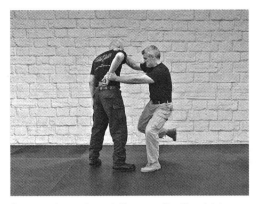 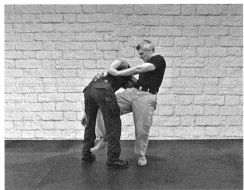

As you close, target the assailant's right arm as he reaches for the weapon. Secure his right wrist with your left hand while simultaneously jolting his right shoulder with your right hand. As you secure his arm and shoulder, knee him in the groin with your right leg.

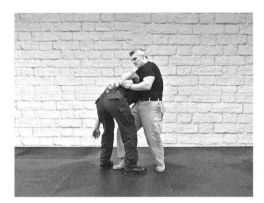 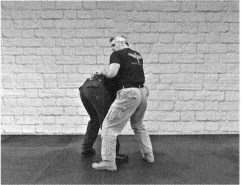

Decisively pin the assailant's right arm to control it while bringing your right arm over the top of his right shoulder to apply Control Hold #6 (kimura). With your free arm, slam the top of your forearm (radial bone) into the crook of the assailant's elbow to fold it, allowing Control #6. Wrench the shoulder forward and up to assert dominant control. Be sure to keep the assailant's shoulder and torso pressed to your body to assert dominant control.

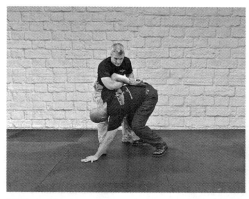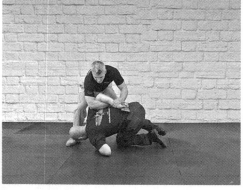

While still asserting dominant control, prepare to drive the assailant to the ground at your two o'clock. As you take down the assailant, be sure to keep his torso close to your torso to prevent any attempt to roll away from you as you drive him to the ground.

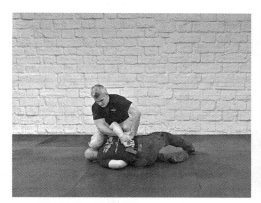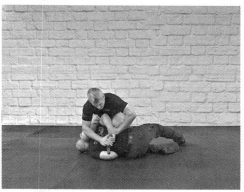

As he drops down, drop with him, landing your left knee at his bent elbow and your right knee on his head, placing all of your body weight on him to control him. Stay on the balls of your feet.

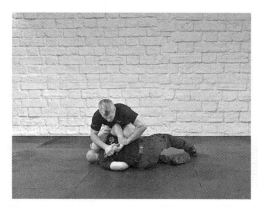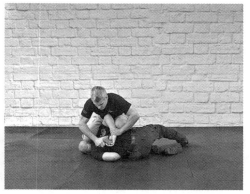

To remove the weapon, keep his left arm pinned with your left arm. With your right hand, secure the barrel to wrench the weapon down and away.

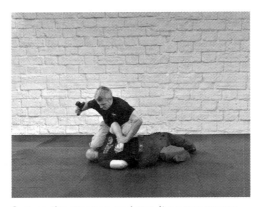

Secure the weapon and use it as necessary.

Note: you do not have to take down the assailant to remove the handgun. Once you have applied Control Hold #6, release your right hand while keeping his arm pinned to your torso with your left arm. Then secure the weapon and remove it from the rear of his waistband. Use the weapon as necessary.

Handgun Defenses from the Front (VIP Protection)

Frontal Handgun Defense #1 with a Companion

Much is written about handgun defenses. Often it is suggested that you should keep your hands raised to feign compliance. But, ultimately, the correct defense simply depends on what position you find yourself in—just be sure to keep your elbows close to your sides. Your goal is to create "zero perception" for the assailant beyond your feigned compliance. In other words, you do not want him to have any indication that you intend to disarm him.

While there is a chance that combatives following the firearm deflection-redirection may knock the assailant out, the goal of these strikes is to stun, short-circuit, and unbalance him enough to allow you to complete the disarming technique. As with all krav maga techniques, if you do not stun the assailant, he will continue to attack—and disarming him will be extremely difficult. Remember, the gun is ergonomically designed for the assailant to hold—not for you, the defender.

Suppose your initial deflection-redirection and body defense have succeeded. Now, as you hit the assailant repeatedly, he is likely to fall or stumble backward, pulling the handgun with him. If you are not properly positioned deep to the deadside, the assailant will yank the handgun back and you will still be in the line of fire. Also, if your combatives have knocked the assailant to the ground but you are improperly positioned, you are also in the line of his kicks, both as he is falling and while he is on the ground. Even if you have jammed the slide, never put yourself in the line of fire. Do not make the mistake of redirecting and counterattacking without properly positioning yourself to the assailant's deadside.

You deflect-redirect the handgun by driving the web of your hand (in between your thumb and index finger) into the front section of the trigger guard. You are punching the handgun away, not slapping or pushing it away. This movement allows your hand to automatically close around the gun deep enough to avoid the muzzle blast (the bullet's exit point on the gun). Additionally, this secure hold provides a grip on the handgun even if it is a short-barreled weapon.

Because the chambered round is likely to fire, you must blade your body to remove it from the line of fire as you simultaneously deflect-redirect the weapon from your body. Properly securing the gun and positioning your body to the deadside is crucial.

Proper Deflecting and Redirecting of Handguns

Many Israeli krav maga imitations and splinter interpretations make the mistake of deflecting-redirecting the gun and attempting to pin it in front of the defender without moving deep to the deadside. Such an errant defense is highly problematic. In other words, the defender does not deflect and *position his torso deep in the assailant's deadside* as the defender puts his full weight on the weapon. This is even more important if the assailant has a two-handed grip, which will obviously allow him more control over the weapon and more strength to resist your disarming technique. Therefore, proper technique must prevail. Deflect-redirect the barrel with all of your weight to maintain dominant control of the weapon and keep your grip very tight to control the barrel.

Krav maga's deflection-redirection method stops the semiautomatic handgun's slide mechanism, preventing a new round from cycling into the chamber or the cylinder of the revolver from rotating. As you deflect and secure the gun, burst forward and sharply jam the gun into the assailant's waist area with the slide of the gun parallel to his body, creating an "elbow kiss." A simultaneous salvo of punches or palm-heel strikes to his head accompanies the deflection-redirection. Your forearm and assailant's gun arm create a "V" as the underside of your forearm presses against the topside of his forearm but not directly on top of his arm.

Your elbow must be behind his elbow for the elbow kiss. Once you have deflected and moved deadside, maintain an elbow kiss while delivering combatives. Be sure to keep your weight firmly pressed down on the barrel of the handgun with your arm flexed to control the weapon. Through your deflection and control arm, place your full body weight on his weapon arm while maintaining deadside position to keep you off the line of fire and reduce his ability to resist—which he is sure to do.

If you decide to disarm an assailant threatening a protectee from the front, gauge the distance between the firearm and your reach to safely control it. It does not matter if the assailant has one or two hands on the handgun grip, and the level of the weapon is not a significant variable, provided you can close the distance and deflect, redirect, and secure the firearm. Note, though, that if the assailant has the gun in one hand, he could blade his body and create a different counterattack angle for you. In addition, with a two-handed grip (depicted below), the assailant can better resist a disarming technique. This underscores the need to move deep into the deadside and to direct strong, debilitating combatives at the head. A two-handed grip leaves his head wide open for your counterattacks.

When the assailant is within your reach, consider your timing. Just prior to launching your disarming technique, lean forward subtly and then punch out with your left hand (assuming the gun is in the assailant's right hand) to deflect and secure the barrel just in front of the trigger guard. Lock out your deflecting-redirecting arm with your full weight on the weapon while transitioning into your body defense to the deadside combined with your simultaneous counterattack.

You can best control the barrel by keeping it parallel to the ground, especially if the assailant attempts to rip it from your grip. Depending both on your height and the assailant's height, you may find the barrel is forced slightly up or slightly down. If you are taller, your controlling grip will force the barrel slightly upward because of the defense's design. If you are shorter, your grip will likely force the barrel downward.

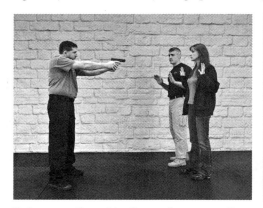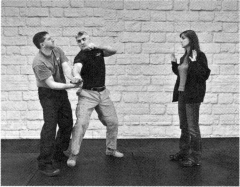

Before any attempt to disarm, keep your elbows at your side and try not to fixate on the weapon. Fixating on the weapon might reveal your intention to disarm the assailant. Slightly shift your weight to the balls of your feet. As you explode forward, deflect and control the handgun close to the trigger guard. When you secure the weapon, lock out your arm while making sure to move deep to the gunman's deadside to create an elbow kiss with your arm flexed. All of your weight bears down on the handgun.

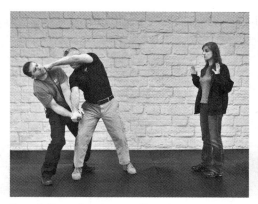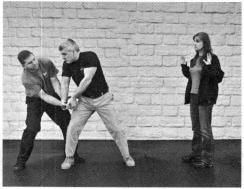

Forcefully strike the assailant in the head using proper body mechanics. You may wish to hit him no fewer than three times to make sure you stun him. To remove the handgun from his grip, maintain your grip on the barrel just above the trigger guard. Move your other arm close to your nearside hip, making sure not to pass any part of your body in front of the muzzle. With your palm up, grab the rear of the handgun above the grip. As you begin to remove the handgun, make sure both of your hands are gripping the gun strongly for control.

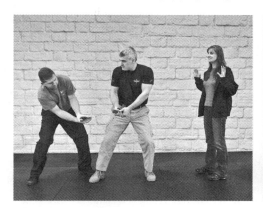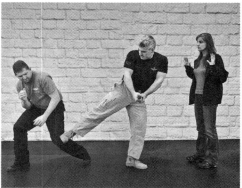

With your right hand rotate or yank the gun back sharply toward your right hip until the handgun grip has rotated a full 180 degrees and is perpendicular to the ground. Pull the handgun back to you by angling the barrel slightly into the assailant to streamline its release from the assailant's trigger finger. This release will likely mangle and break his trigger finger. You may also jolt him with your nearside shoulder while tucking your chin to knock him backward, facilitating the release. To further debilitate him, deliver a strong side kick to his nearside knee.

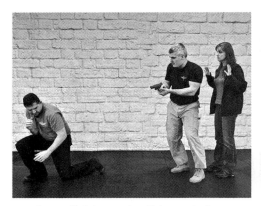 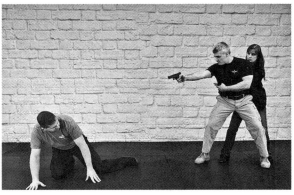

Immediately create distance between yourself and the assailant, seating the magazine and racking the weapon to place it into battery if you are familiar with the type of weapon. Place yourself in front of your companion and secure your companion's arm while maintaining a strong firing platform.

Frontal Handgun Defense #2 with a Companion

This double-handed disarming technique redirects the gun and simultaneously removes it from the assailant's grip.

A defender may use Frontal Defense #2 if Defense #1 would redirect the line of fire toward a bystander. Defense #2 can also be used to counter the combined strength of a two-handed handgun grip. Another scenario is if you are with a companion who would be in the line of fire if you use Frontal Defense #1. Or you may simply feel more comfortable with this defense.

The handgun is once again in the assailant's right hand or held by both hands. (Note again that it does not matter if the assailant has one or two hands grasping the handgun.) You will redirect the firearm opposite to the direction in Frontal Defense #1. This technique is very powerful and focuses on the weakest part of the assailant's grip, the inner palm, rather than trying to work against his combined finger clutch strength.

There are a few similarities between Frontal Defenses #1 and #2. As with Frontal Defense #1, when an assailant threatens you from the front, if you must disarm him, gauge the distance between the firearm and your reach. If the assailant is within your reach, consider your timing.

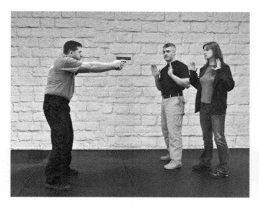
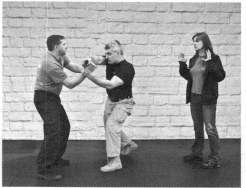

Before any attempt to disarm, keep your elbows at your side and try not to fixate on the weapon. Fixating on the weapon might reveal your intention to disarm the assailant. Slightly shift your weight to the balls of your feet. As you explode forward, deflect and control the handgun close to the trigger guard. As you secure the weapon, lock out your arm while making sure to move deep to the gunman's deadside to create an elbow kiss with all of your weight bearing down on the weapon. Using a subtle forward lean on the balls of your feet, punch out with your right hand in conjunction with bursting forward. Step toward the weapon to deflect and secure the handgun by the barrel while blading your body. Use your left hand to simultaneously secure and yank down sharply on the wrist of the assailant's gun arm. Keep your left thumb beside your palm in a cupping motion. The simultaneous movement of punching and yanking down helps to create a scissoring motion to dislodge the handgun. Be sure to use a simultaneous body defense to move off the line of fire.

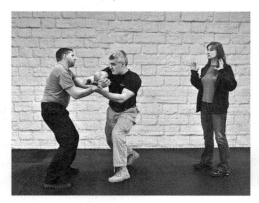
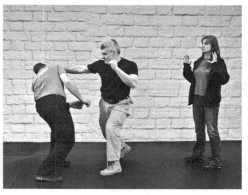

Forcibly punch the handgun through and away from the assailant's grip, jarring the wrist of his gun arm to allow you to punch the weapon out of his grip. Use the handgun as a cold weapon to stun the assailant (or you may deliver a straight kick with whichever leg is best positioned to do so).

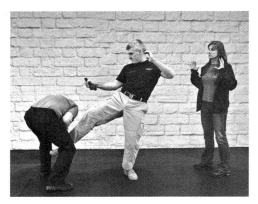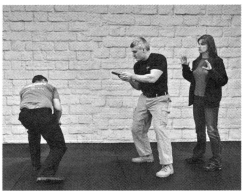

Kick the assailant in the groin with your right leg to further debilitate him. Immediately create distance between yourself and the assailant, seating the magazine and racking the weapon to place it into battery. Place yourself in front of your companion and secure your companion's arm while maintaining a strong firing platform.

If for some reason you do not succeed at punching the handgun out of his hand(s), relentlessly press your counterattack, making sure to stay out of the line of fire. The assailant will likely retract the handgun to pull it away from you. Keep your hands firmly in place and move with his pullback while executing lower body combatives, including knees and straight kicks while moving to the assailant's deadside. *Do not under any circumstances let go of the handgun.* Be careful that the assailant does not hit you with an inadvertent head butt as a result of your lower body combatives lurching him forward. Continue your lower body combatives while maintaining strong control of the handgun.

VIP Frontal Long-Gun/Submachine Gun Defenses

Long-gun or submachine-gun (SMG) defenses from the front are similar in concept to handgun defenses but different in execution because of the firearm's length.

Defending against a long-gun or SMG threat utilizes the core krav maga principle of simultaneous weapon deflection-redirection and body defense movement combined with counterattacks. A distinct difference between a long-gun or SMG design and a handgun is the firearm's length, especially if the long gun or SMG has an extended stock. Certain SMGs such as the Uzi pistol might need to be defended using the handgun defenses covered previously. Shotguns are also included in the long-gun category for the purposes of our discussion. Keep in mind, however, that a shotgun's discharge creates a wider berth of danger as the cone of fire scatters.

Krav maga's long-gun/SMG and bayonet-type defenses adapt to threats at different heights. The following three frontal defense variations are also used to thwart a bayonet-type attack. Whichever defense you use, be sure to remain clear of the muzzle while controlling it. A semiautomatic or automatic long gun or SMG will continue firing as long as the gunman activates the trigger and the ammunition supply lasts. An automatic weapon can discharge thirty-plus rounds in just a few seconds. Keep in mind that these rounds also endanger third parties. Long-gun/SMG disarming techniques do not interfere with the firing mechanism as some of krav maga's handgun defenses do.

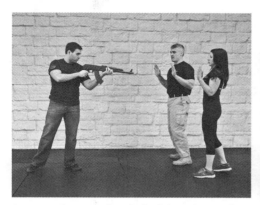
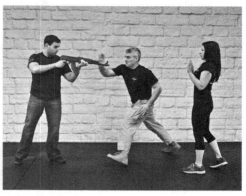

As you raise your hands in feigned compliance, keep your elbows at your side and try not to fixate on the weapon. Fixating on the weapon might reveal your intention to disarm the assailant. Slightly shift your weight to the balls of your feet. As you explode forward, deflect-redirect the long gun with your right hand as you prepare to loop your left arm around the long gun for control.

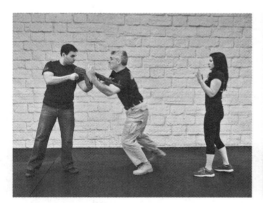
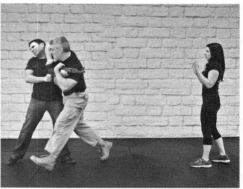

As you close on the assailant, wrap your left arm around the barrel and into the crook of your elbow. As you secure the long gun in the crook of your elbow, deliver an over-the-top elbow strike to his head. You can also add knee strikes to further stun and debilitate him.

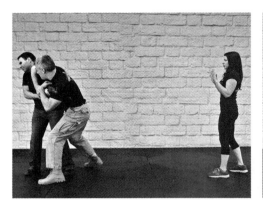
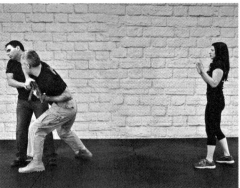
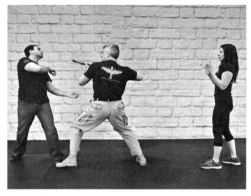

To remove the long gun from his grip, reach for the weapon's rear pistol grip. (Note that this weapon has a retracted stock; if the weapon did not have a retracted stock, you would reach for the front of the stock.) Wrench the long gun out and away by pulling up on the bottom of the pistol grip or the gunman's cupped hand. Rotate your body sharply away to secure the weapon. After removal, use the weapon as necessary.

Neutralizing a Threatening Gunman or Active Shooter, Rear Approach

When there is no "bullet to the head" or other option but to attempt disarming an armed third party threatening others, or in an active-shooter situation, it is best to use a gross motor movement to surprise the gunman from the rear. A tackle coupled with a *kosoto gake* (forward trip) variation works well against a stationary or moving gunman. As noted, the tackle is one of the most effective takedown techniques. Like other combatives, the tackle's power derives from hip and leg explosion.

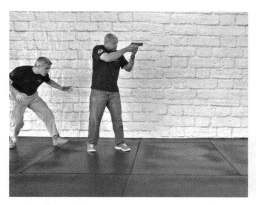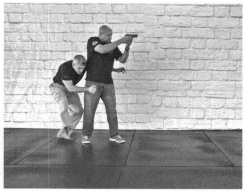

Focus on driving your shoulder just below your adversary's hips or midsection, with your head to one side of his torso. Bull your neck and keep your face up. Just prior to contact, sink your hips with a wide leg base to explode through your adversary. This is similar to rising from a squat, but you will also churn your legs for momentum.

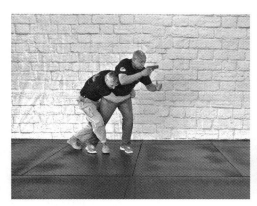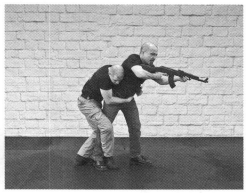

Wrap your arms around the gunman's waist or hips to drive him forward. Our natural reaction when being driven forward is to put our hands out in front to deal with the impact of falling face first, so he *may* drop the weapon, whether a handgun or long gun. The tactic is the same for either weapon.

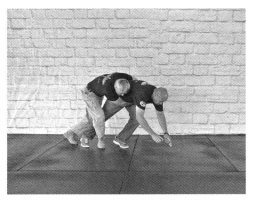

Secure him tightly on the way down, keeping your head buried, and prepared to let go just as the gunman collides with the ground.

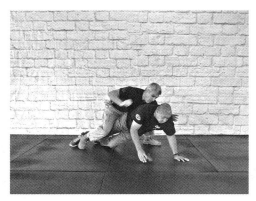
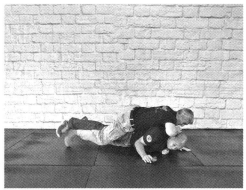

If the gunman does not release the handgun, you must again quickly take his back while pounding him with one arm and securing the weapon with a good portion of your weight on it.

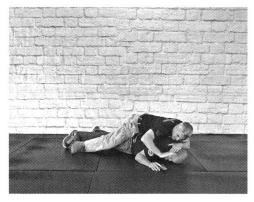
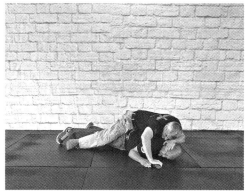

If he continues to hold the handgun, secure the barrel with your right arm to wrench it from his grip.

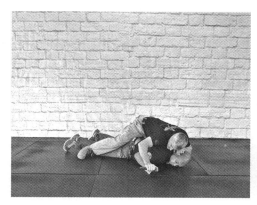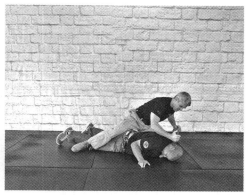

With a firm grip, rotate the handgun's barrel down and away and use it as a cold weapon. Get up, create distance, and place the weapon back in battery.

Active-Shooter Takedown if the Gunman Releases the Handgun

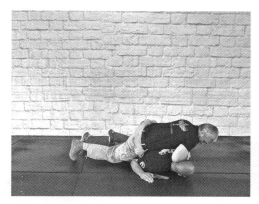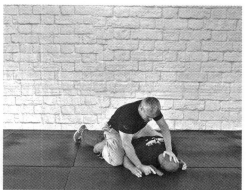

If the gunman releases the weapon as he is driven into the ground, continue to take his back. Administer strong combatives to his head and neck using forearm, elbow, punches, or palm heel strikes, perhaps followed by a stomp as you get up quickly after neutralizing him. (Note: when disarming a long gun, you may be able to choke him with the weapon. But when disarming a handgun, beware of choking him if he maintains possession, since he can simply shoot you in the head as you attempt the choke.)

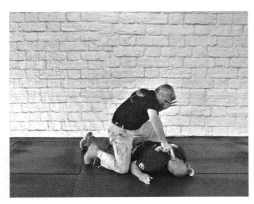 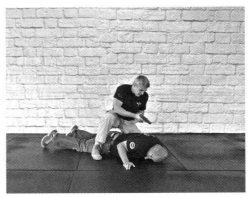

Secure and use the handgun as necessary in a cold weapon capacity.

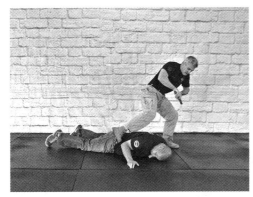 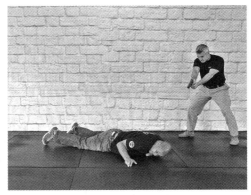

Get up and create distance. Prepare the weapon and train it on the assailant.

Neutralizing a Threatening Gunman or Active Shooter, Rear Approach, Handgun Option

When there is no other option but to attempt disarming a third party threatening others with a firearm, or an active shooter, you may wish to disarm the gunman from the rear using a specific weapon-removal technique combined with tai-sabaki. You must approach as silently as possible, aware that your approach could cast a shadow the gunman might see or he could hear your approach. This takeaway requires great timing and precision. Against a right-handed gunman, your final step before attempting the disarming technique should be with your left foot to enable the tai-sabaki takeaway.

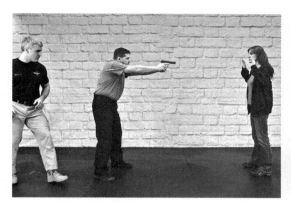 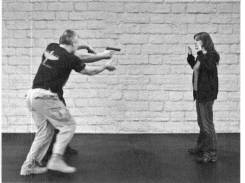

In this handgun-disarming technique, as you step with your left foot positioned parallel to the gunman's legs, secure his right arm with your left arm above his wrist, using an underhand grip. Your right hand secures the handgun just in front of the trigger guard.

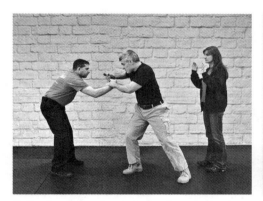 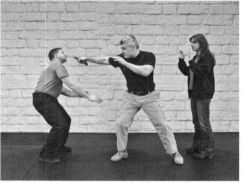

Both of your hands must simultaneously clamp down on the gunman's right upper wrist and the handgun. Immediately after clamping down, step forward with your right leg to punch the handgun toward the gunman's upper body. Sharply wrench the handgun away from the gunman, punching the barrel into his face or neck by using the power of the tai-sabaki movement. After forcing the gun 180 degrees, dislodge the weapon from his grip by yanking it out and away to release it from his trigger finger.

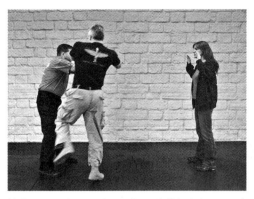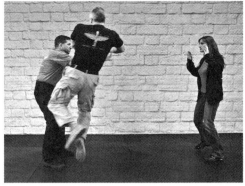

Note: an advanced version of this takeaway incorporates a simultaneous scissors kick as you punch the weapon away. As you step forward with your left leg, quickly step with your right leg. As your right foot touches the ground, jump up with the right leg to deliver a straight right kick to the assailant's groin.

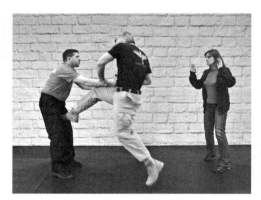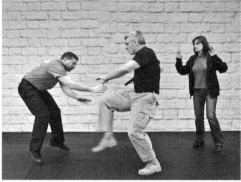

Kick the assailant in the groin while keeping a secure grip on both his arm and the handgun. Use the jumping kick's momentum to help dislodge his grip on the handgun.

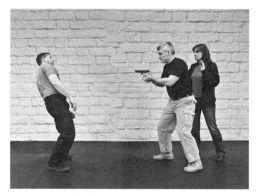

Keep in mind that if the gunman pulls the trigger as you confiscate the weapon, you will likely force a stoppage, rendering the handgun inoperable. Let the continued momentum of the tai-sabaki create distance as you tap and rack the weapon to put it back into battery.

Neutralizing a Threatening Gunman or Active Shooter, Rear Approach, Long-Gun Option

A defense similar to the previous option of disarming an assailant with a handgun is used for a long gun. (The gunman is right handed.)

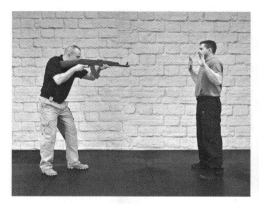
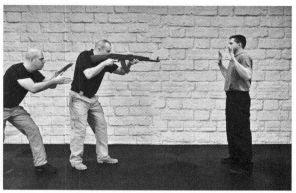

Step with your left foot positioned parallel to the gunman's legs.

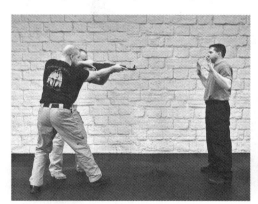
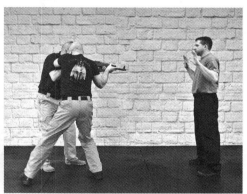

As you step forward with your right leg, secure the stock with your left arm by reaching over the top of the gunman's elbow as your right hand, using an underhand grip, secures the long gun at the foregrip. Both of your hands should clamp down simultaneously on the long gun. Immediately after clamping down, step forward with your right leg to wrench the barrel down toward the ground and then rotate it toward the gunman's torso.

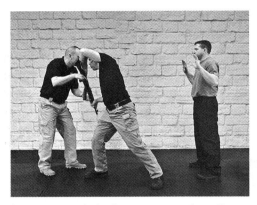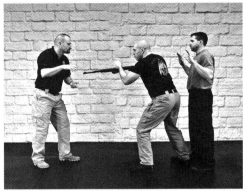

Sharply wrench the long gun away from the gunman by directing the barrel down and away and then into him by using the power of the tai-sabaki movement. After forcing the long gun down and away and then 180 degrees, dislodge the weapon from his grip by yanking it out and away to release it from his trigger finger.

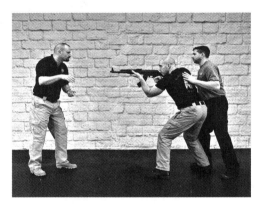

Redirect the long gun at the assailant, placing the former hostage behind you. Keep in mind that if the gunman presses the trigger as you confiscate the weapon, the long gun (unlike a handgun) will remain in battery and continue firing until it runs out of ammunition, though there is a possibility of dislodging the magazine. If it is a magazine-fed weapon, let the continued momentum of the tai-sabaki create distance as you tap the magazine and rack the weapon to ensure it is in battery. Note: for photo purposes, the distance between the gunman and defender is abbreviated and would be considerably greater as the defender moves the hostage to safety while also maintaining a safe distance from the assailant.

Note: if the long gun's stock is lodged under the gunman's armpit, you must adapt the technique by forcing the barrel up and away and then into the gunman's torso.

Note: an advanced version of this takeaway incorporates a simultaneous scissors kick as you wrench the weapon up and away.

Neutralizing a Gunman Threatening with a Handgun to a Hostage's Head, Rear Approach

When there is no "bullet to the head" or other option but to attempt disarming a third party threatening a hostage with a firearm, you may wish to disarm the gunman from the rear using a specific weapon-removal technique combined with tai-sabaki. Once again, you must approach as silently as possible and aware that your approach could cast a shadow the gunman might see. This takeaway requires great timing and precision. Against a right-handed gunman, your final step before attempting to disarm must be with your left foot to enable the tai-sabaki takeaway.

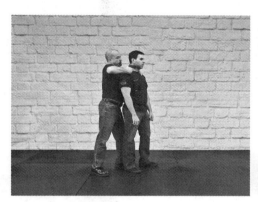 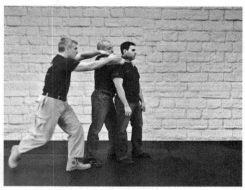

Step with your left foot positioned parallel to the gunman's legs and secure his right arm with your left arm above his wrist while your right hand, using an underhand grip, secures the handgun just in front of the trigger guard. You must do this precisely as the handgun barrel must be diverted decisively away from the hostage and toward the hostage taker.

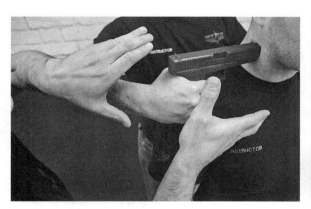 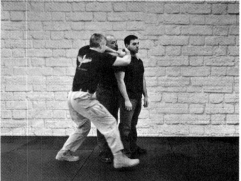

Both of your hands must clamp down simultaneously on the gunman's right arm.

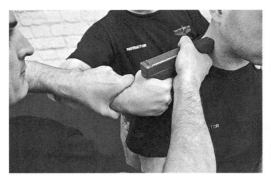 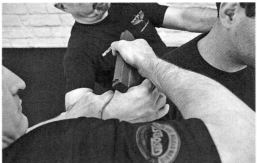

Redirect the barrel toward the assailant.

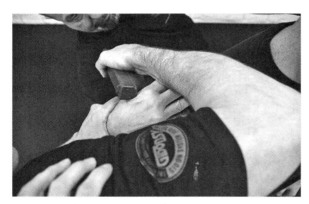 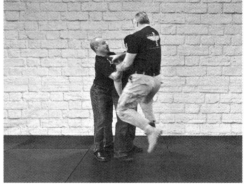

Immediately after clamping down, step forward with your right leg to punch the handgun in the direction of the gunman's head. Note that the advanced version of the depicted takeaway incorporates a simultaneous scissors kick to the *hostage's* groin to force the hostage to the ground as you punch the weapon away. (The tactic is designed to put the hostage on the ground, allowing you to have a clear field of fire at the assailant.) As you step forward with you left leg, quickly step with your right leg. As your right foot touches the ground, jump up and on the right leg to deliver a straight kick to the *hostage's* groin.

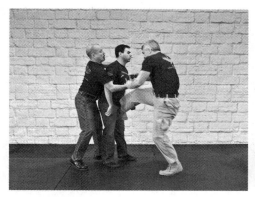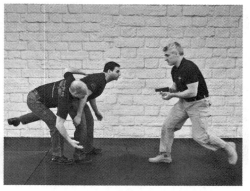

As you kick the hostage in the groin, wrench the handgun away from the gunman, directing the barrel into him by using the power of the tai-sabaki movement. After forcing the handgun 180 degrees, dislodge the weapon from his grip by yanking it out and away to release it from his trigger finger.

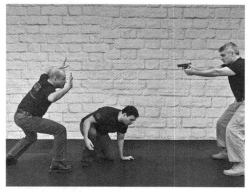

Secure the handgun and create distance. Again, keep in mind that if the gunman pulls the trigger as you confiscate the weapon, you will likely interfere with the slide's correct functioning, forcing a stoppage. Use the continued momentum of the tai-sabaki to create distance as you tap and rack the weapon to put it back into battery.

Neutralizing a Third Party Threatening with a Hand Grenade, Rear Approach

An assailant might hold a hand grenade in a threatening manner. The grenade may or may not have the safety pin removed. Until identified, the defender should assume the grenade is primed and ready to explode once the spoon or detonation mechanism is released. The crucial difference with a primed grenade, of course, is that you do not want to hold on to it but rather dispose of it quickly. If the grenade is not primed and the pin is intact, of course, you will confiscate it after felling and neutralizing the assailant.

Similar to all other krav maga defenses, the assailant must be debilitated and the weapon safely removed and controlled. After incapacitating the assailant with low-line kicks to the groin combined with Cavalier #1 and followed by a heel stomp to the head, the best way to dispose of the grenade—if it cannot be thrown to a safe location—is by placing it under the assailant's torso to absorb the brunt of the detonation. Move quickly and decisively with economy of motion. Take a direct line to the assailant while remaining out of his line of vision.

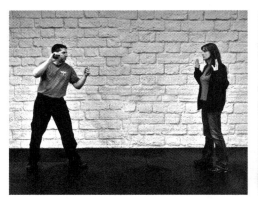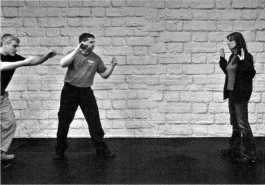

A terrorist is holding a third party hostage with a grenade. Step with your left foot positioned parallel to the terrorist's legs.

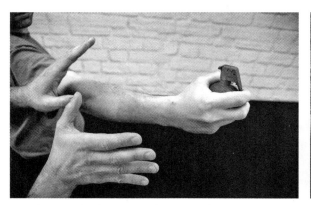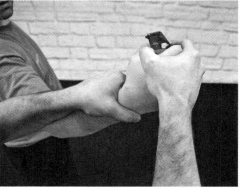

Secure his right arm with your left arm above his wrist while your right hand, using an underhand grip, secures the grenade using a "knuckles to knuckles" grip. (In essence, you are performing Cavalier #1 as covered in many previous defenses.) As you step forward with your left leg, quickly step with your right leg.

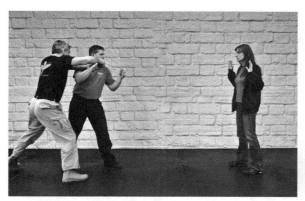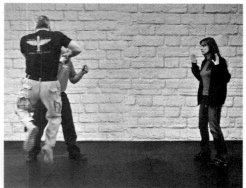

As your right foot touches the ground, jump up and on the right leg to deliver a straight kick to the assailant's groin while keeping a secure grip on both his arm and on his right hand and grenade.

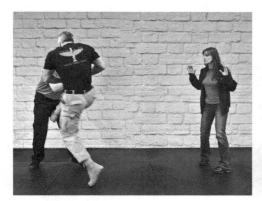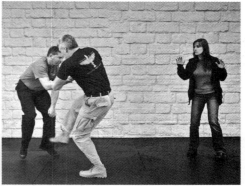

Use the jumping scissor kick's momentum to help dislodge the grenade from his grip, though the tactic can be performed with out a jumping scissor kick, instead simply using Cavalier #1.

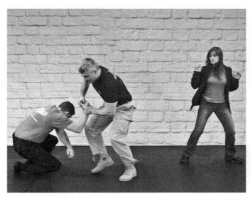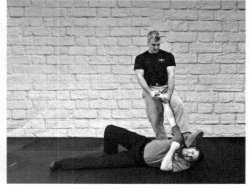

After delivering the kick, continue with the Cavalier #1 modification and take the assailant to the ground. Kick him in the head with your heel, optimally targeting his temple. You must injure and stun him with a forceful, targeted kick. At this stage it is paramount that you immediately recognize if the pin is in or out of the grenade. If the pin is intact, the spoon will not release to detonate the grenade. You can then safely maintain possession and *not* perform the following steps.

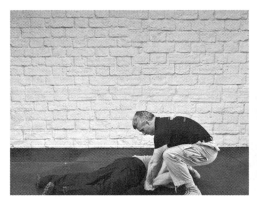 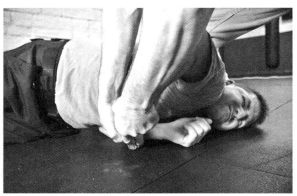

As noted, if the pin is out and the spoon has released, you must kick the assailant in the head with your heel—preferably in the temple—at least once to neutralize him. After you kick him in the head, if you cannot safely throw the live grenade away, you must insert the grenade underneath the terrorist for him to absorb the imminent blast. To do this, torque his wrist using a modification of Cavalier #1 to force his right side slightly off the ground. This creates a gap between his body and the ground. Force his arm under his body to jam the grenade into this gap.

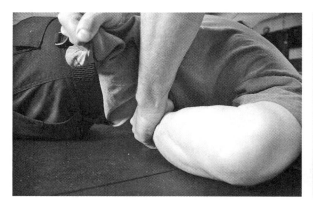 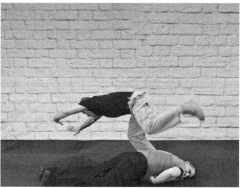

Execute a proper high roll. Using your arms as a spring to soften the fall, turn your head and tuck it to the side, rolling diagonally across your back.

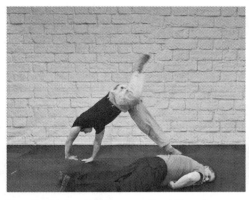 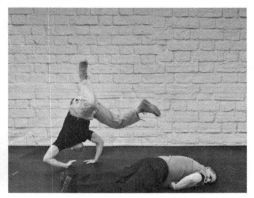

Use the high roll to escape the kill radius.

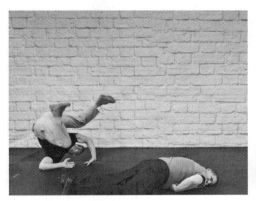 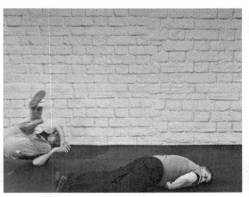

Complete the roll and fall into position with your feet facing the adversary. The soles of your shoes will take any blast fragments sent your way.

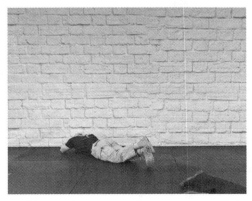

Cover your head and ears with your forearms and open your mouth to alleviate the impending blast concussion.

CHAPTER 9

Firearm Retention and Professional Kravist Weapon-Defense Drills

Sidearm Retention

Sidearm retention is a foremost concern for law enforcement, military, and other lawfully armed personnel. For sidearm retention, before the assailant can grab the defender's weapon, krav maga uses basic deflection-redirection defenses with a 180-degree hip pivot to take the gun-side hip away while simultaneously striking the assailant or creating distance.

If the assailant successfully grabs the defender's holstered weapon, the simultaneous defense and attack principle dictates that with a typical level 3 or 4 retention holster, the defender must secure the weapon with preferably his forearm or, if necessary, his hand or by pressing against the top rear of the slide while delivering combatives with the free arm, legs, and possibly head butts. In the case of a tactical thigh rig, both hands may be needed to secure the weapon, necessitating knee strikes or kicks while turning the gun leg away from the assailant and tucking the chin to protect the throat.

Sidearm Retention, Twelve O'Clock Threat

This defensive option intercepts someone attempting to grab your firearm from your twelve o'clock.

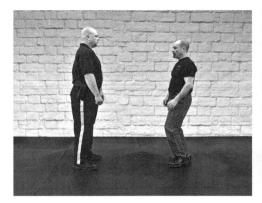 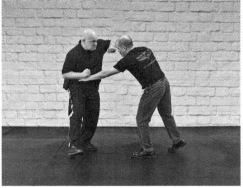

With your nearside (weapon-side) arm, use a modified forearm chop/rotation to deflect the assailant's reaching arm.

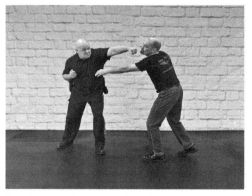

As you ward off the assailant's incoming arm, pivot 180 degrees, using tai-sabaki. At the same time, use your opposite arm to deliver a strike to the assailant's head. As you do so, immediately create distance for a higher use-of-force option or, alternatively, close on the assailant to detain him.

Sidearm Retention, Three O'Clock Threat

This defense, by design, is similar to previous sidearm frontal retention techniques.

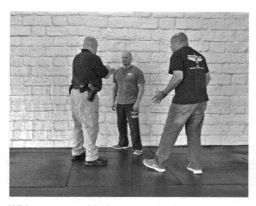
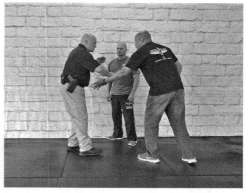

With your nearside (weapon-side) arm, use a modified forearm chop/rotation to deflect the assailant's reaching arm.

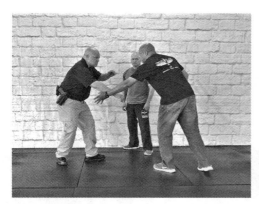
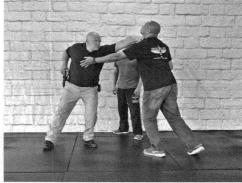

As you ward off the assailant's incoming arm, pivot 180 degrees, using tai-sabaki. As you pivot, use your opposite arm to deliver a strike to the assailant's head.

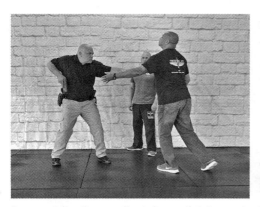
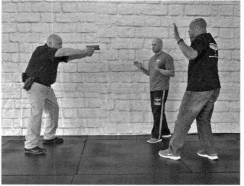

As you strike the assailant, immediately create distance and deploy your sidearm.

Sidearm Retention, Three O'Clock Threat (Thigh Holster Variation)

This defense, by design, is similar to previous sidearm frontal retention techniques.

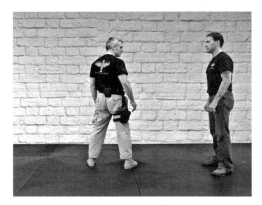 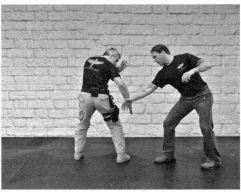

With your nearside (weapon-side) arm, use a modified forearm chop/rotation to deflect the assailant's reaching arm.

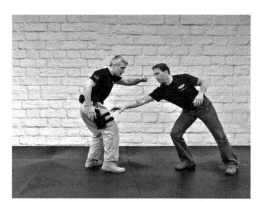 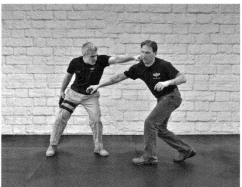

As you ward off the assailant's incoming arm, pivot 180 degrees, using tai-sabaki. At the same time, use your opposite arm to deliver a strike to the assailant's head. As you strike the assailant, immediately create distance and deploy your sidearm.

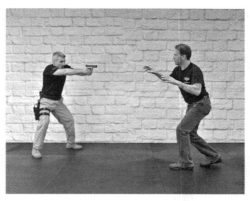

Maintain your distance to control the situation with a clear field of fire.

Sidearm Retention, Six O'Clock Threat

This defense is appropriate if an assailant is able to "get the drop" on you or approach you from the rear undetected and attempt to grab your sidearm.

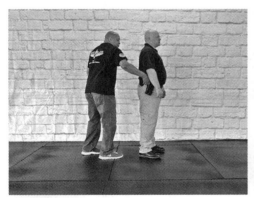 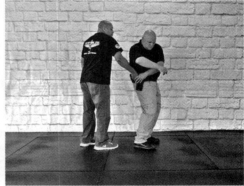

Defend initially with your nearside (weapon-side) arm by clamping down on, or delivering a compact elbow strike to, his reach hand. If the assailant succeeds in grabbing your pistol grip, use your left hand to clamp down hard, smashing his thumb or the top of his hand. As you ward off the assailant's incoming arm, pivot 180 degrees, using tai-sabaki.

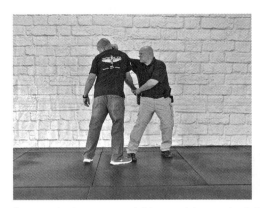 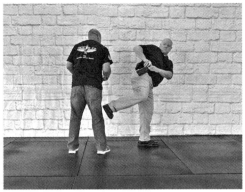

As you pivot, use your right nearside arm to deliver a strike to the assailant's head.

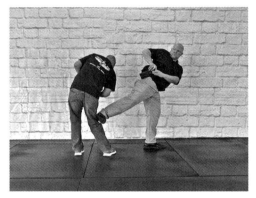

You may further debilitate him with a side kick to his knee. After you stun the assailant, immediately create distance for a higher use-of-force option or, alternatively, close on the assailant to detain him.

Sidearm Retention, Six O'Clock Threat (Alternative #1)

If an assailant is able to "get the drop" on you or approach you from the rear undetected and attempt to grab your sidearm, another defensive option is to clamp down with your weapon-side arm and wheel around to strike him in the head.

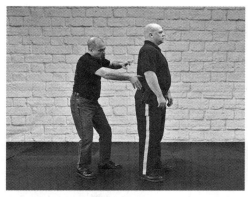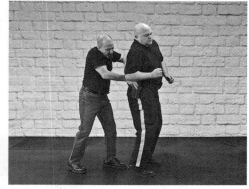

Clamp down with your weapon-side arm on top of the holster or the assailant's hand.

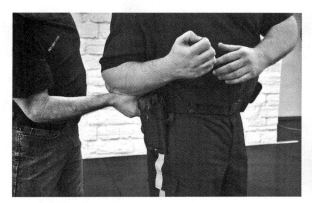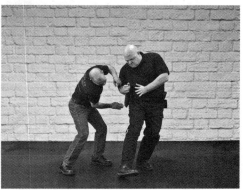

Continue to clear his hand from your holster by turning clockwise to face the threat. Note: another option (not depicted) is to clamp down with your weapon-side forearm and turn your head over your other shoulder to club the assailant with your free arm. As you club him, pivot away to gain distance and release his hand from your holstered weapon.

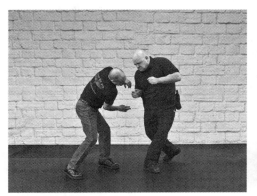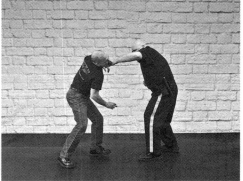

As you clear the threat, continue to take a tai-sabaki step while simultaneously delivering a strike to the assailant's head.

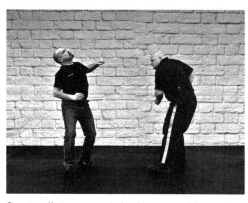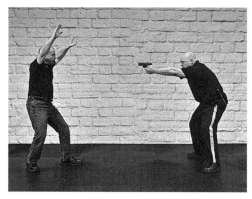

Create distance and deploy your sidearm to control the threat or, alternatively, close on the assailant to detain him.

Sidearm Retention, Six O'Clock Threat (Alternative #2)

This third option is similar to the previous defense. Use it if an assailant "gets the drop" on you or approaches undetected from the rear and attempts to grab your sidearm. Clamp down and wheel around to strike him in the head.

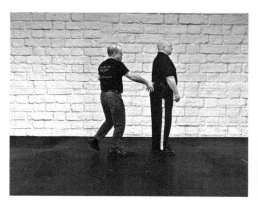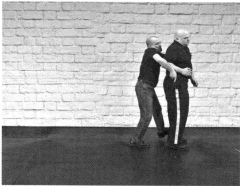

Clamp down with your weapon-side arm on top of the holster or the assailant's hand.

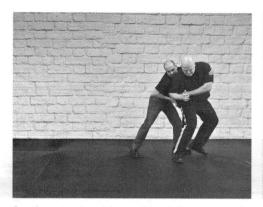 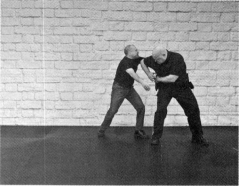

Continue to clear his hand by delivering an elbow to his midsection, solar plexus, or chin. Create distance and deploy your sidearm to control the threat or, alternatively, close on the assailant to detain him.

Deployed Sidearm Retention, Twelve O'Clock Grab Attempt

If you have your handgun deployed and, for whatever reason, do not want to shoot an assailant attempting to grab it, a weapon-retention option is to rotate the weapon in a *small* semicircle to avoid his grasp while simultaneously using the handgun as a cold weapon. You may also, of course, simply strike him directly in the face with the weapon to preempt his grab attempt.

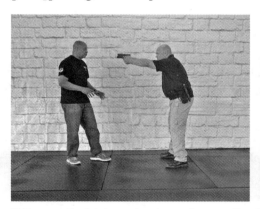 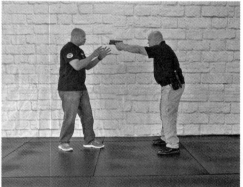

If the assailant takes advantage of a negative-five situation to close the distance on you and reach for your deployed sidearm, you may thwart his attempt by rotating your weapon counter-clockwise in a tight circle (usually preferable for right-handed shooters) or clockwise (usually preferable for left-handed shooters).

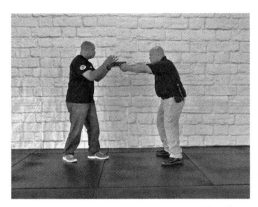
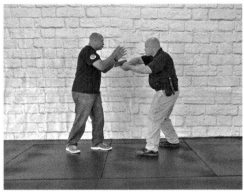

As you rotate the weapon to prevent him from grasping it, continue with your tight loop to use it as a cold weapon to attack the assailant's head. Note: you can use your two-handed firing grip or release your weak-side hand to better control the firearm as a cold weapon.

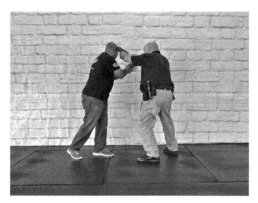
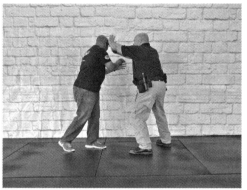

Forcefully strike the assailant in the head with the barrel. An alternative strike is to remove your support hand and use it to support the barrel strike to the assailant's head. Continue with retzev combatives or create distance for a clear field of fire.

Deployed Sidearm Retention, Twelve O'Clock Threat (Assailant's Hands on Your Weapon)

If the assailant is able to place his hands on your sidearm, a strong retention tactic is to pull your elbows close to your torso while stepping forcefully with your nearside leg in front of the assailant to make him relinquish his grip. If for whatever reason you do not want to shoot an assailant who is able to place his hands on your weapon, a weapon-retention option is to step forward strongly while raising your elbow, which simultaneously points the barrel down and away.

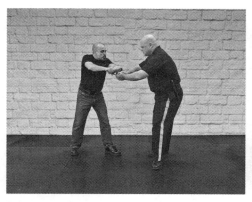
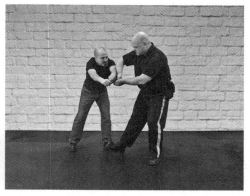

Raise your right elbow and step with your right leg forward to "punch" your shoulder into the assailant to facilitate removing his grip. Jolt the assailant with your nearside shoulder to create further separation.

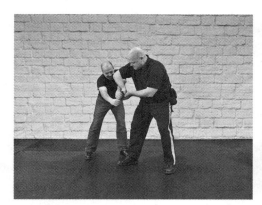
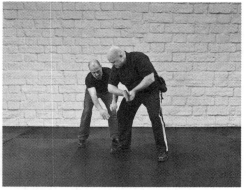

Use the handgun as a cold weapon or use a lower-body combative to debilitate the assailant. As you release his grip, immediately go on the counteroffensive by using the handgun as a cold weapon to strike the assailant in the head. Or use lower-body combatives to create distance and discharge the firearm into the assailant—as legally justified and necessary. The key is not to let the assailant attack or take your back.

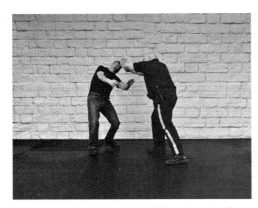 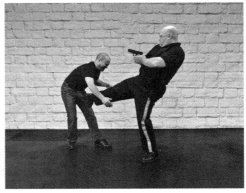

Finish as necessary with additional combatives such as the front kick depicted, or create distance to control the situation and use the firearm as needed.

Note: you could also step forward with your left leg and pull the weapon back to face the assailant and not turn your back. The advantage of this is that you have the barrel still facing the assailant. However, the nearside leg stepping forward is depicted because it is a stronger option for a smaller person against a much larger, possibly more powerful assailant and is also used similarly for long-gun retention in a similar situation.

Long-Gun or Submachine Gun Weapon Retention, Twelve O'Clock Kick Option

Instinctively, a defender usually will not willingly let go of or give up his weapon. Obviously, your first optimum reaction is to shoot the assailant. The following long-gun defenses assume you cannot take the initial shot.

Krav maga, as with most of its other tactics, builds on this instinct to maintain or wrest control away from the assailant. The defense, similar by design to most krav maga defenses, parallels an unarmed "bear hug" defense with the arms free.

If the assailant attempts to grab the long gun from the rear while the defender's arms are raised with the weapon in either the low or high ready rifle positions, the defender will naturally take a step forward or back. Importantly, from a low ready rifle position, if the assailant grabs the barrel, the defender can also drop to one knee, which will usually point the barrel directly at the assailant's pelvis or midsection, allowing an effective shot. The direction of motion, in turn, usually depends on if the assailant is driving the defender forward or back. In one of krav maga's few counterintuitive movements, the defender is encouraged to move *with* the assailant rather than resist him. Long-gun or SMG retention, with or without a sling, uses the simple concept of turning the assailant's force against him as he attempts to wrest the weapon away.

By using leverage and footwork combined with barrel rotations, the defender can disengage the weapon from the assailant's grip. Against a right-hand grab of the muzzle, it is recommended to rotate the barrel or muzzle clockwise while stepping forward. This is followed by a rifle combative or low-line kick, or by stepping backward to free the weapon and possibly shooting the assailant. If the assailant grabs the barrel with his left hand, rotate the barrel clockwise while stepping forward with combatives. Or step backward to disengage and then shoot. The long gun or SMG is also turned trigger side in to break the assailant's grip. At the same time, you turn the magazine in to the assailant, clearing the way for kicks and knee counterstrikes.

Alternatively, if your long gun is slung and the assailant has grabbed it, you may close on the assailant to collar-tie clinch him while transitioning to a secondary weapon or to attack his head. This could include a thumb gouge to his same-side eye or a forceful manipulation of his neck. Move with the assailant as he pulls at your weapon to harness his momentum and your momentum and seize control of his head. For the clinch, even though he may have your primary weapon in his hands, you must account for his ability to fight back and possibly seize your secondary weapon, including an edged weapon.

The collar-tie clinch allows you to control the assailant's head and keep him close, but be aware of the possible countermeasures he may use. The goal is to get one of your weapons on line while exerting maximum control of the assailant or, if possible, to create enough separation to deploy your primary or secondary firearm. Note: of course, a defender can use weapon-retention or cold combatives and then go "hot."

Long-gun or SMG retention, with or without a sling, uses the simple concept of turning the assailant's force against him as he attempts to wrest the weapon away. By moving in the direction of the weapon pull, the defender's momentum increases the power and effectiveness of the strikes.

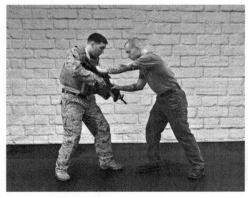 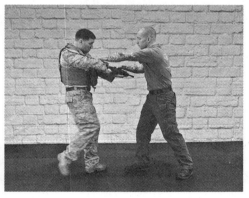

Move in the direction in which the adversary pulls the weapon, harnessing his momentum and your momentum against him. This will enhance the power and effectiveness of your lower-body strikes.

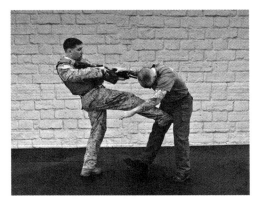

It is important to rotate your long gun's magazine housing into the assailant, as this provides you with a much stronger grip and clears the magazine for your lower-body combatives. (Note: krav maga uses the technique of rotating the magazine housing into the opponent when using a disarming technique against him.) Immediately create distance with a clear field of fire.

Long-Gun or Submachine Gun Weapon-Retention Rotations

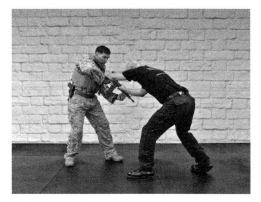
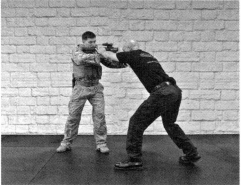

The long gun's grips are obviously designed for the shooter to maintain control. By forcefully rotating the weapon clockwise, the assailant will have a difficult time holding on to it.

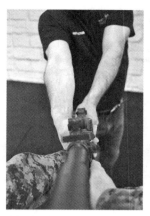

Beginning position.

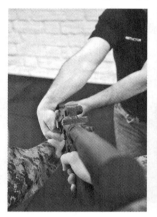
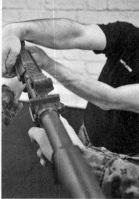

Rotation 2.

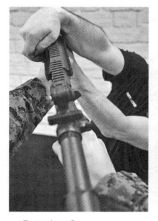
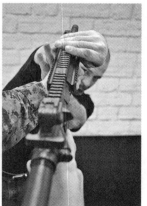

Rotation 3.

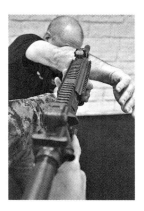

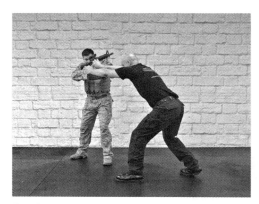
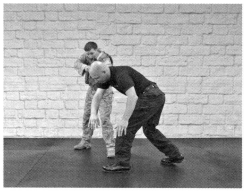

Continue to rotate the long gun clockwise to clear it and create a clear field of fire.

Twelve O'Clock Grab When an Assailant Wrenches the Slung Weapon Away into Clinch and the Defender Has a Sidearm

Your instinct, most likely, is not to let go of your weapon. Yet if the assailant succeeds in grasping it and wrenching it partially or fully from your grip, a weapon-retention option—provided your weapon has a sling and you have a functional sidearm—is to use a one-armed, crown-of-the-head clinch to secure the assailant while deploying your sidearm to shoot him. This tactic is obviously only available to those who have a sidearm, although the defender could also deploy a blade to counterattack.

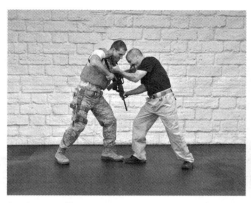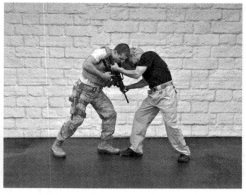

As the assailant pulls your weapon, keep it secured with your shooting hand, using the sling for weapon-retention reinforcement. Clinch the back of his head with your left arm. Similar to the previous defense, it is important to harness the assailant's momentum as he pulls backward in an attempt to pull your long gun away.

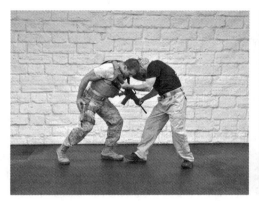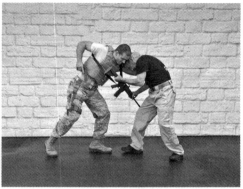

Once you have the assailant firmly clinched with your left hand, transition to your handgun.

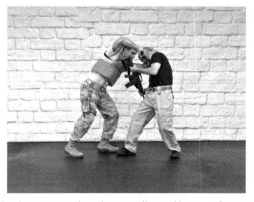

Use a point-shoot method to neutralize the assailant. Note: a few methods of shooting the assailant may be used, and it is up to one's individual preference.

Long-Gun Weapon Retention While Defending Takedown Attempts

Long-Gun Strikes against Tackle Attempts

Against a rear tackle attempt, the defender (using correct timing and distance) has a few options depending on his recognition of the incoming attack and its angle. Fortunately, an operator's equipment and weapon at the ready position can make it difficult for an assailant of average size to wrap his arms around the defender.

Twelve O'Clock Tackle Attempt

Against a front tackle attempt, the defender, using correct timing and distance, has a few options—besides shooting the onrushing assailant:

1. Thrust the muzzle into the assailant's face or throat.
2. Sidestep the attack and slash down on the assailant's head with the muzzle.
3. Extend the foregrip or magazine into the assailant's carotid sheath or neck by using a subtle sidestep while maintaining a strong body posture and position to thwart the attack.
4. Sprawl with the weapon raised high, maintaining your weight on the assailant's neck to bury his head into the ground and continue your counterattacks.

Note: it is also possible to deliver a preemptive straight rear kick, a knee, or front side-kick to the assailant's head if he is crouched, or to his body if he is more upright, before he can close on you to attempt a takedown. But a long gun is a highly effective tool, and it is better for the defender to keep his legs firmly planted on the ground with his weight on the balls of his feet.

Twelve O'Clock Modified Sprawl

If you do not have time to shoot him or perform one of the previously discussed options, you may have to use a modified sprawl.

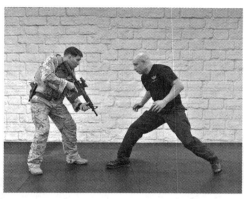

From the low ready rifle position, as the assailant drops down in his front takedown attempt, angle your long gun with the muzzle to the ground. From a high ready rifle position, you would use your forearms and the weapon as an "A" frame or wedge as you sprawl.

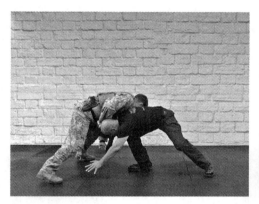 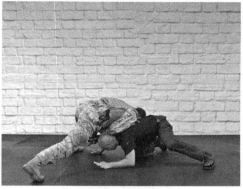

As he closes on you, sprawl your legs backward with a wide base. Drive your weight into him. Try to remain on the balls of your feet rather than on the sides of your feet to facilitate your ability to get up quickly.

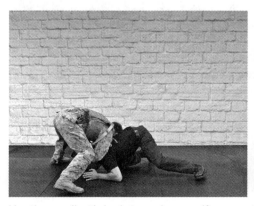 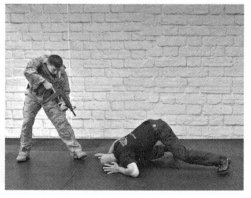

Use the assailant's body to push yourself up, create separation, and use your long gun as necessary.

Long-Gun Retention Twelve O'Clock Tackle

This tactic is effective when an assailant is able to successfully come underneath your weapon, wrapping his arms around you to take you down.

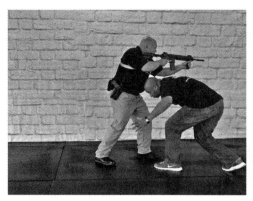 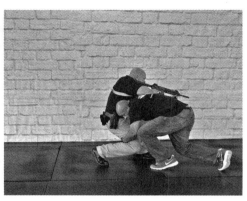

You must fall break effectively with your back while maintaining solid control of your long gun.

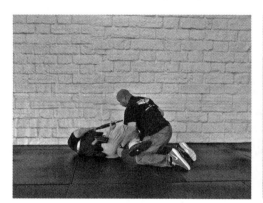 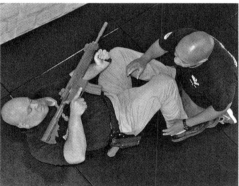

As you fall break to the ground, immediately position your topside foreleg against the assailant to prevent him from mounting you while also allowing you to jolt him back to create separation. As you position your topside leg, try to place your bottom-side heel against his hip or thigh for the Z guard.

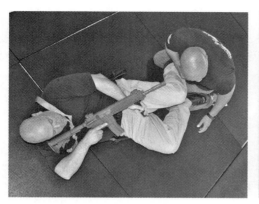
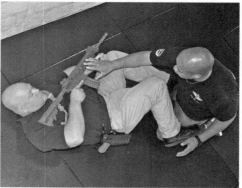

Control the assailant with your legs and bring your long gun online.

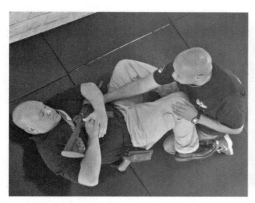
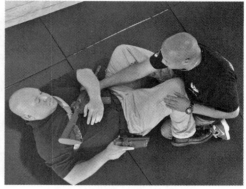

If the assailant continues to reach for your long gun, clamp it tight to your torso and transition to your sidearm (or an edged weapon). (Note: if you do not have a side arm, extend your legs to kick the assailant and create separation to allow you to use your long gun.)

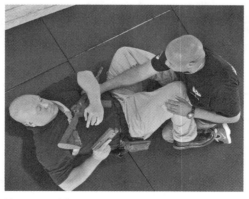

Use your sidearm as necessary.

Long-Gun Three O'Clock Retention

With early recognition, you may use clockwise rotations to defend against an assailant's attempt to wrest your weapon from you. This is similar to the twelve o'clock retention technique.

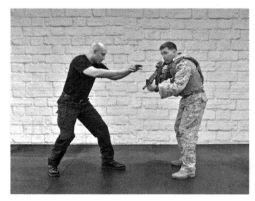 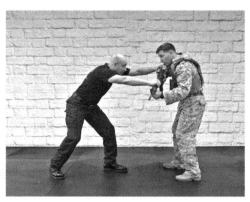

The long gun's grips are obviously designed for the shooter to maintain control. By forcefully rotating the weapon clockwise, the assailant will have a difficult time holding on to it.

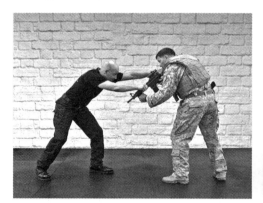 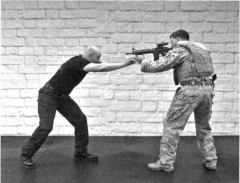

Continue to rotate the long gun clockwise to clear it and create a clear field of fire.

Long-Gun Four to Five O'Clock Retention

This is similar to the six o'clock retention. With early recognition, the defender may deliver a butt strike to the assailant's head or, if the assailant is crouched, a rear heel kick to the assailant's head and, if more upright, to the torso. If the defender's recognition is late and he goes facedown, he must land (fall break) correctly and then instantaneously raise his rear knee (assuming he is a right-handed shooter) to transition 180 degrees to the foreleg brace position to keep the assailant momentarily at bay. Next he must disengage from the assailant and establish a solid shooting platform to use his primary or secondary weapon. Note: it is also possible to deliver a straight rear kick if the assailant is approaching from the liveside or front sidekick if the assailant is approaching from the deadside. In either case, the target is either the head, if he is crouched, or the body, if he is more upright. Note again, however, a long gun is a highly effective tool, and it is better for the defender to keep his legs firmly planted on the ground with his weight on the balls of his feet.

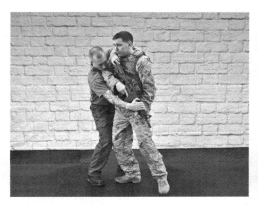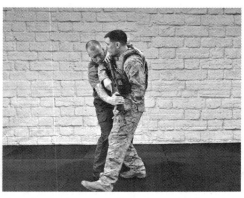

The long gun's grips are obviously designed for the shooter to maintain control. By forcefully rotating the weapon clockwise, the assailant will have a difficult time holding on to it. Note: as an alternative, you can also deliver a short sidekick to the assailant's right or left knee.

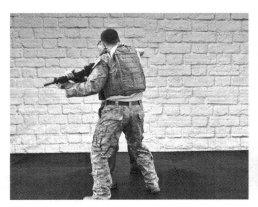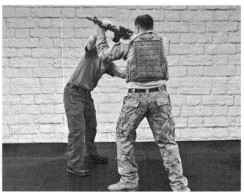

Continue to rotate the long gun clockwise to remove it from his grasp.

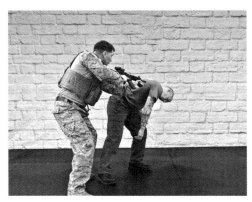

Create a clear field of fire.

Long-Gun Four to Five O'Clock Retention When Tackled

If you are ambushed from the rear with a tackle, you must recover quickly by falling correctly and then immediately turning to face the assailant.

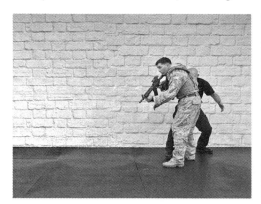
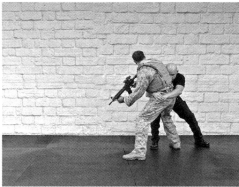

On first contact, as the assailant wraps his arms around you, swivel your head and begin to turn your front into him.

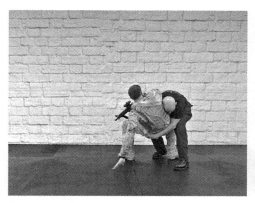
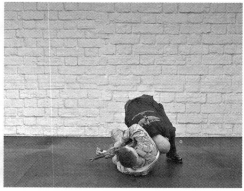

As you continue to turn but are driven back, lower your support arm to lessen the impact. Be sure to bend and angle both your wrist and arm slightly to avoid injuring them as your arm absorbs the combined weight of you and your assailant.

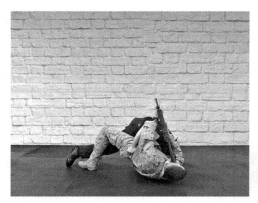
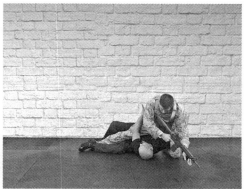

Land on your back and continue to turn into him. As soon as you make contact with the ground, secure your weapon with your support arm again and bridge into the assailant. Note: if you are so combat laden that you cannot easily turn into the assailant to pin him, you may, as an alternative, remain on your back, pivot your body 180 degrees (not depicted), and turn your legs toward him to ward him off for a stable firing platform.

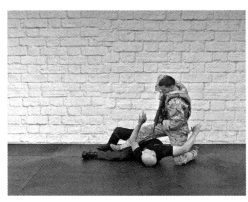

Create separation, if possible landing on top of him or to his side to bring your long gun to bear.

Long-Gun Six O'Clock Retention

The attack here comes from behind, your six o'clock. With early recognition, the defender may deliver a butt stroke to the assailant's head or, if the assailant is crouched, a rear heel kick to the assailant's head, and if more upright, to the torso. Note again, however, a long gun is a highly effective tool, and it is better for you to keep your legs firmly planted on the ground with your weight slightly on the balls of your feet. If the assailant does succeed in closing on you from your six o'clock, react instantaneously by turning into him before he can secure his arms around you or your weapon.

Harnessing the assailant's momentum obviously takes training. And if the defender is caught unaware, the assailant will move him in one direction or the other; the defender must simply flow with it. If the assailant drives the defender forward, the defender will step forward. Depending on which way the defender steps—forward or to the rear—the defender's front or rear leg will be "loaded" as it takes his weight. When one leg is loaded, the other leg gains more freedom of action, such as to administer a punishing knee or kick. The weight transfer also allows the defender to pivot off the line of attack. As the defender pivots, he may use the long gun for a close-quarters battle point-shoot option or in a cold-weapon capacity.

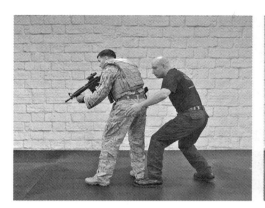
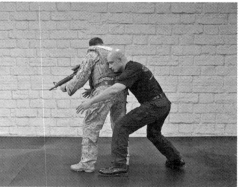

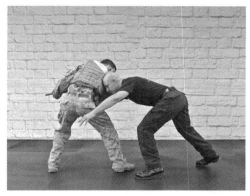

As the assailant makes contact, take a natural step forward to move with the initial jolt. Try, however, not to place all of your weight on your front leg. As you step, begin to take a step with your forward leg to the outside off the line of attack.

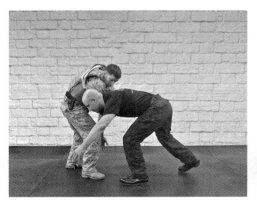
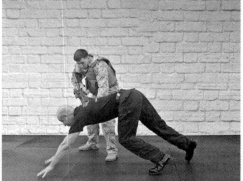

Turn away from him, beginning to break contact and separate.

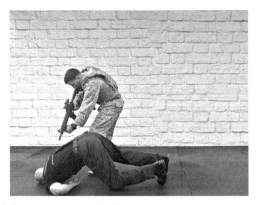

Create separation and bring your weapon to bear.

Long-Gun Retention Six O'Clock Tackle Attempt with the Defender
in the Ready Position: Reverse Sprawl

If an assailant is able to approach you from your six o'clock position, you must build your defense on his forward momentum carrying you forward. If you recognize the impending attack just as he is about to latch onto you, you may perform a reverse topside or "face-up" sprawl, landing on the assailant's head or upper torso. The additional weight of your armor, load-bearing vest, or helmet will aid in this. Quickly get up or transition 180 degrees to keep his front pinned to the ground, allowing you to continue counterattacks from an advantageous position.

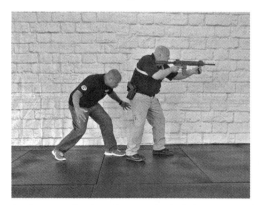 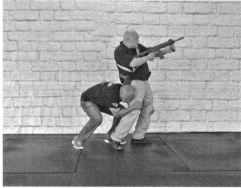

As the assailant makes contact, take a natural step forward with your rear leg or both legs to move with the initial jolt. Let both of your legs move forward.

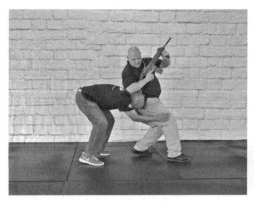 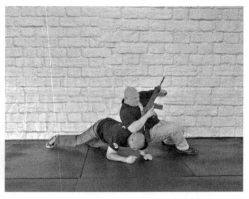

As you step forward, let your weight fall back, centering it on his neck and shoulder as he drives underneath you. "Reverse sprawl" with him and allow your legs to move forward slightly while driving your weight into him.

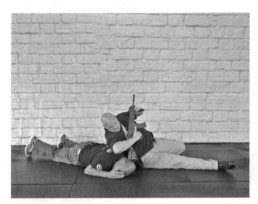 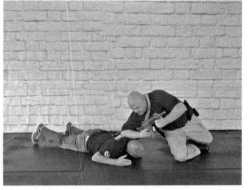

Use the butt of your long gun or your elbow to smash him in the head as you both descend. Get up immediately.

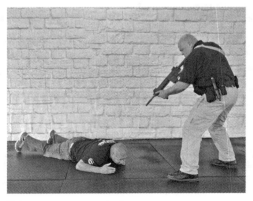

Bring your weapon to bear.

Long-Gun Retention Six O'Clock Tackle Attempt with the Defender in the Ready Position: Turn into the Foreleg Brace Position

If the assailant succeeds in ambushing you from your six o'clock position, move forward with the tackle to break the fall and immediately transition into the default foreleg brace position.

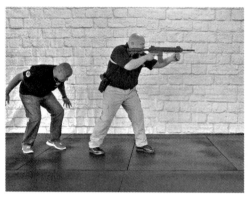
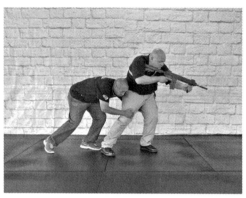

As the assailant makes contact, step forward to move naturally with his initial jolt.

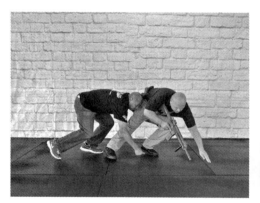
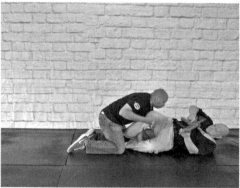

Land and fall break correctly, extending your forward arm to help absorb the impact with the ground. Be sure to angle your lead hand and wrist properly not to injure yourself on impact as you break your fall. Immediately on touching the ground, turn onto your back. As you do so, raise your topside knee to instantly transition to the foreleg brace position.

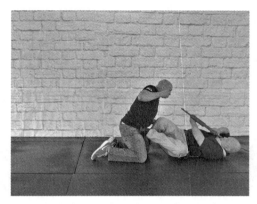

As you turn, insert your bottom leg's foot against the assailant's hip to keep the assailant momentarily at bay. Bring your weapon to bear and disengage from the assailant while establishing a solid shooting platform to use your primary or secondary weapon.

Long-Gun Retention against a Nine O'Clock Grab Attempt

If your long gun is slung and your arms are down, the assailant may or may not be able to get his arms around you. It depends on a few variables, including your recognition and reaction to his incoming grab, how wide you are with your gear, and how long the assailant's arms are. In any event, you must focus on not allowing the assailant to secure any kind of hold on your long gun. Similar to the previous weapon-retention tactics, by denying the assailant any control, you can counterattack and then create space to place your long gun online. Immediately turn to face the assailant to use the long gun in a hot- or cold-weapon capacity.

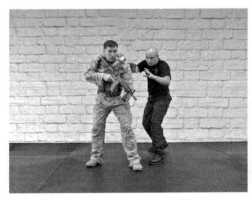 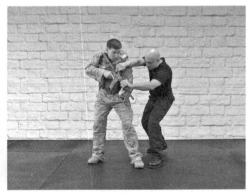

The long gun's grips are designed for you to maintain control. The assailant will have a difficult time holding on to it if you forcefully rotate the weapon clockwise.

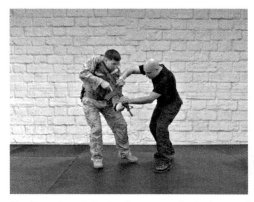 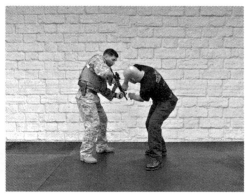

Continue to rotate the long gun clockwise to clear it.

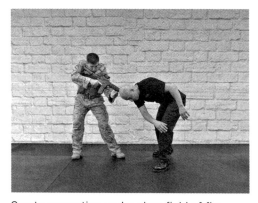

Create separation and a clear field of fire.

Use of Force

Use of Force and Law Enforcement,
by Sergeant First Class Mick McComb, Ret.

My opinions on the use of force (UOF) are based on twenty-five years of service with the New Jersey State Police. For ten years I was assigned to the NJSP Training Bureau in roles including lead academy instructor; assistant unit head for the Firearms and Self-Defense Training Unit; use of force instructor; and lead defensive tactics instructor, including training recruit, advanced, and in-service members. I authored and revised self-defense lesson plans, appeared in US District Court and deposition on behalf of the State of New Jersey regarding use-of-force litigation matters, and served within the Office of Professional Standards (formally IAB) as a supervisor and investigator, specifically in use-of-force investigations.

Law enforcement personnel are often faced with difficult decisions, perhaps none more difficult than using coercive force. The primary objective for law enforcement when engaged in a use-of-force incident is to restrain and control while utilizing an "objectively reasonable" amount of force. The often asked, debated, and second-guessed law enforcement question is how much force is necessary, required, or acceptable? One point requires emphasis. Generally, there is no reason for law enforcement officers (LEOs) to strike a suspect in the head outside of a deadly force encounter. The following terms require discussion:

Excessive use of force: This term can be described as using more force than a reasonable person would deem reasonable and necessary.

Unnecessary or unreasonable amount of force: This term refers to law enforcement personnel who utilize force where a reasonably prudent and well-trained police officer would not. If law enforcement personnel are accused of utilizing too much force, accountability for the incident(s) will include, but not be limited to, possible discipline for violating department policy, agency rules and regulations violations, internal investigation complaints, possible criminal charges, and civil lawsuits.

Today many UOF encounters involving law enforcement officers and the public are captured on video from police cruisers, body cameras, cell phones, or other electronic devices. These encounters often look completely different from the reality of the event and do not tell the entire story. One's perceptions, lack of knowledge, understanding of the law, department policy, the constitutional standard and relevant standards, biases, subsequent rush to judgment, media pressure, politics, administrative incompetence, outside influences, and overreactions as well as other factors will determine one's interpretation of the event.

A myriad of considerations underpin reasonably objective use of force. Circumstances; application of force; force options; training; experience; department policy; attorney general guidelines and the constitutional standard set forward in Graham v. Connor, 1989; along with other relevant factors are taken into account when evaluating a use-of-force incident. Attempting to physically control an unwilling, uncooperative individual who is either passively or actively resisting arrest is one of the most dangerous, difficult, and stressful situations faced by law enforcement.

Training (or lack thereof), skill level, physical conditioning, fatigue, strength, physical and emotional control, attitude, decision-making skills, roadway conditions, time of day, uniform restrictions, equipment, and other factors including but not limited to the number of officers present all play vital roles during in determining the objective reasonable use of force. Each UOF incident is independent of another. Each should be considered as a unique, independent set of circumstances. However, this often is not the case.

The UOF standard was set by the Supreme Court case *Graham v. Connor*, 1989. The court advised lower courts to ask three main questions regarding use of force:

- What was the severity of the crime law enforcement believed the subject committed?
- Did the subject present an immediate threat to law enforcement or the general public?
- Did the subject resist arrest or attempt to escape?

Additional criteria, as noted previously, are also considered when evaluating the *Graham v. Connor* standard and its implementation.

Under the Constitution's Fourth Amendment, law enforcement officers are permitted to utilize what is known as "objectively reasonable force." This standard applies when a LEO seizes a free person. Under this standard, LEOs may choose from their force options and employ force that is objectively reasonable. Force can and should be used by LEOs based on the suspect's actions, capabilities, and under the totality of the circumstances.

Law enforcement personnel must realize and understand that during any UOF confrontation it is the subject who *chooses* to resist a LEO's authority and control. As a result, the subject prolongs the confrontation and, in most instances, determines when UOF will cease by freely *choosing* to stop resisting and comply. Until the subject submits to the LEO's control, the application of force will not end; however, the force utilized must be objectively reasonable. LEOs must also realize that good verbal communication skills, a well-written and detailed report, good judgment, sound decisions, knowledge of the law, department policy, and proper documentation are all essential factors when assessing a UOF incident. Once again, *it is imperative that law enforcement personnel realize that in a lawful seizure of a person, in most instances, the subject, in fact, controls or determines many aspects regarding UOF.*

- The majority of the time, the subject initiates the UOF incident.
- The subject determines when force will cease (by ceasing resistance and complying). Note: this is where many LEOs exceed the objectively reasonable use of force standard by failing to de-escalate or, when appropriate, terminate their UOF.

Once the subject stops resisting and complies, LEOs must restrain and control, ratcheting down any use of force to possibly none at all, other than applying restraints. When a subject is restrained with handcuffs, leg shackles, or both, LEOs must recognize that the use-of-force incident is over. It is unacceptable, unauthorized, and against accepted police policies, practices, procedures, and relevant standards to strike a subject under these circumstances.

Use-of-Force Standard: Objective Reasonableness

The reasonableness of a LEO's use of force is partially based on the circumstances *known* by the LEO at the exact moment force was used. The standard of objective reasonableness only applies to the use of force upon a "seized free person." Certain factors dictate the reasonableness standard. They are, in order of priority, as follows:

- **Imminent threat to LEO(s) or others:** Is the suspect an imminent threat to law enforcement or others?
- **Actively resisting arrest:** Is the subject actively resisting arrest, and if so how? What are the subject's actions, what threat does the subject present, and how does it make the officers feel? Law enforcement officers can choose among their "force options," as long as it is deemed to be objectively reasonable.
- **Circumstances are tense, uncertain, and rapidly changing:** If so, law enforcement may escalate and justify their level of force by choosing within their force options.
- **Severity of crime:** The more severe the crime committed by the subject, an increase of force can be justified.

Summary of Force Options

- **Constructive:** The use of a law enforcement officer's authority to exert control over the suspect. Command presence, uniform, and voice inflection.
- **Physical:** Physical bodily contact with the suspect, normally utilized to make an arrest or meet another law enforcement objective. Hands, fists, and feet.
- **Mechanical:** Device that employs less-than-deadly force. Baton, oleoresin capsicum spray, flashlight, and canine.
- **Enhanced mechanical**: Conductive Electronic Device (CED). Depending on a department's policy and state-authorized guidelines, this option is normally between mechanical and deadly force.
- **Deadly:** Force used in an encounter in which law enforcement personnel reasonably believe there is a substantial risk of causing death or serious bodily harm.

Severe Threat Level and Factors

The more severe the threat posed to law enforcement officers, the more force they can justify. Let us look at some of these factors:

- **Totality of circumstances.** The objective, reasonable use of force implemented by law enforcement will be judged on the "totality of circumstances" known by the officer at the time force was used.
- **Intrusiveness.** Law Enforcement use of force *does not* have to be the least intrusive option available. Choosing from any of their "force options" (objectively reasonable).
- **Objectivity.** Refers to what others would logically believe or conclude. Would a reasonably prudent and well-trained law enforcement officer who knows the law believe what the officer did was acceptable?
- **Moment of use.** Law enforcement's use of force will be judged regarding *the moment force is used*.
- **Constitutional standard.** The constitutional standard is the Fourth Amendment, *Graham v. Connor*, 1989. This standard states: "The right of the people to be secure, in their persons, homes, papers, and effects, against unreasonable searches and seizures, shall not be violated, and no warrants shall issue, but upon probable cause, supported by oath or affirmation, and particularly describing the place to be searched, and the persons or things to be seized."

Note: the information contained within is not meant to be a substitute for legal advice and the writer is not an attorney. It is highly recommended that any law enforcement officer who might be involved in litigation or use of force consult an attorney as well as a use-of-force expert.

Remember there is a distinct difference between law enforcement and military krav maga training. Not everyone understands or honors this important separation. A common mistake is to teach law enforcement techniques for military purposes. To be sure, there can be overlap, but military training, when taught correctly, focuses on maiming or terminating an enemy combatant. As noted, we only teach lethal-force applications to vetted personnel through our military training programs.

Biographies

Grandmaster Haim Gidon

Grandmaster Haim Gidon, tenth dan and Israeli Krav Maga Association president, heads Israeli krav maga (Gidon System) from the IKMA's main training center in Netanya, Israel. He was a member of krav maga founder Imi Lichtenfeld's first training class in the early 1960s. Along with Imi and other top instructors, Haim Gidon cofounded the IKMA. In 1995 Imi nominated Haim as the top authority to grant first-dan krav maga black belts and up. Haim represented krav maga as the head of the system on the professional committee of Israel's National Sports Institute, Wingate. Grandmaster Gidon, whose professional expertise is in worldwide demand, has taught defensive tactics for the last thirty years to Israel's security and military agencies. He is ably assisted by some of the highest-ranked and most capable krav maga instructors in the world, including Ohad Gidon (sixth dan), Noam Gidon (fifth dan), Yoav Krayn (fifth dan), Yigal Arbiv (fifth dan), and Steve Moshe (fourth dan). More information is available at www.kravmagaisraeli.com.

Senior Instructor Rick Blitstein

Rick Blitstein is one of a few hand-picked individuals who traveled to Netanya, Israel, in 1981 to complete an intensive krav maga instructors' course. Under the watchful eye of krav maga founder Imi Lichtenfeld, Israeli experts taught Rick for the purpose of introducing krav maga to the United States. Imi and Rick formed a very close bond and spent much time training together in both Israel and the United States. For much of the past twenty years, Rick has worked in the field of private and corporate security, teaching and using krav maga in real-life situations. A member of the IKMA and recognized as a senior black-belt instructor, Rick is committed to the proper expansion of the system in the US and around the world. Rick sent his student David Kahn to train with the IKMA for instructor certification.

H. C. "Sparky" Bollinger

H. C. "Sparky" Bollinger is a retired US Marine Corps officer and a United States Judo Association board member with more than thirty-five years of martial arts experience. Sparky holds multiple high-level rankings in several disciplines and systems, including a fourth dan in Japanese jujitsu from the USJA. Professionally, Sparky has trained senior hand-to-hand combat and defensive tactics instructors for the US Marine Corps, British Royal Marines, British Royal Navy, FBI Academy, FBI Hostage Rescue

Team, DEA Academy, New Jersey State Police Academy, Tennessee Department of Corrections SWAT teams, and a host of other agencies.

Instructor/Photographer Rinaldo Rossi

Black-belt instructor Rinaldo Rossi began his krav maga training in 2001 and his advanced training with David Kahn in 2006. Rinaldo completed his instructor certification with Grandmaster Haim Gidon in both the United States and Israel. Rinaldo is one of only a few Americans to complete Grandmaster Gidon's certification course in Israel. Rinaldo instructed at several prestigious locations, including the Naval Special Warfare Advanced Training Command, Marine Corps Martial Arts Center of Excellence (MACE), US Army Combatives School, and the FBI Academy. Rinaldo is responsible for the national rollout of Israeli krav maga in the United States with Don Melnick in coordination with the Israeli Krav Maga Association.

Resources

Asian World of Martial Arts
9400 Ashton Road
Philadelphia, PA 19114
(800) 345-2962
www.awma.com

Aries Fight Gear
(800) 542-7437
www.punchingbag.com

Mancino Mats
1180 Church Road
Lansdale, PA 19446
(800) 338-6287
www.mancinomats.com

Authentic Israel Army Surplus
P.O. Box 31006
Tel Aviv 61310
Israel
US Local Phone: (718) 701-3955
Toll Free Number: (888) 293-1421
Israel: (972) 3-6204612; Fax: (972) 9-8859661
www.israelmilitary.com

To read more about krav maga and its history:

Israel Defense Forces
Homepage: krav maga.idf.il

Israeli Special Forces Krav Maga
Homepage: www.ct707.com

Israeli Krav Maga Association (Gidon System)
Homepage: www.israelikrav.com and www.kravmagaisraeli.com

Index

About the Author

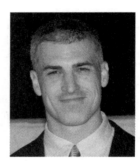

David Kahn, IKMA United States chief instructor, received his advanced black-belt teaching certifications from Grandmaster Haim Gidon and is the only American to sit on the IKMA Board of Directors. The United States Judo Association also awarded David a fifth-degree black belt in combat jujitsu. He has trained all branches of the US military, the Royal Marines, as well as federal, state, and local law enforcement agencies. David has instructed at many respected hand-to-hand combat schools, including the Marine Corps Martial Arts Center of Excellence (MACE), US Army Combatives School, a Naval Advanced Training Command, and the FBI and New Jersey State Police Academies. He is a certified instructor for the State of New Jersey Police Training Commission. David is regularly featured in major media outlets, including *Men's Fitness, GQ, USA Today, Los Angeles Times, Washington Post, New Yorker, Penthouse, Fitness, Marine Corps News*, Armed Forces Network, *Special Operations Report*, and Military.com. He previously authored the books *Krav Maga, Advanced Krav Maga*, and *Krav Maga Weapon Defenses*. He also produced the *Mastering Krav Maga* DVD series, volumes I, II, III, and IV, and volume I supplement: *Defending the 12 Most Common Unarmed Attacks*, along with the *Mastering Krav Maga Online* program. *Mastering Krav Maga Online* includes 333 lessons, or more than twenty-six hours of online lessons, covering approximately 90 percent of the krav maga civilian curriculum. Please visit: www.masteringkravmaga.com.

David and his partners operate several Israeli krav maga training centers of excellence. For more information, contact info@israelikrav.com or the following:

Israeli Krav Maga US Main Training Center
860 Highway 206
Bordentown, New Jersey 08505
(609) 585-MAGA
www.israelikrav.com

Israeli Krav Maga Association (Gidon System)
PO Box 1103
Netanya, Israel
www.kravmagaisraeli.com